THE EVERYTHING®
GUIDE TO LIVING
GLUTEN-FREE

Dear Reader,

Since you have picked up this book, chances are you, or someone you love, is about to begin living gluten-free. In the beginning, the thought of eliminating bread and wheat can seem impossible. I wrote this book to help ease you through that transition. I promise—things will get easier.

I was diagnosed with celiac disease in 2008 after living with unexplained symptoms for more than fifteen years. Thankfully, doctors are beginning to realize that some seemingly random illnesses may be connected to the gluten in our diet, and are suggesting a gluten-free diet to their patients more frequently.

After being diagnosed with celiac disease, I knew that it would lead to a lifelong change in my diet. Rather than sulking over the foods I could no longer have, I decided that I would find a way to continue enjoying my favorite flavors by figuring out how to make them gluten-free. Dealing with well-meaning friends and family and attending social events were other challenges to overcome. These pages contain everything I have learned since beginning my gluten-free diet. My hope is that you will benefit from my experience as you begin living your gluten-free life.

Jeanine Friesen

Welcome to the EVERYTHING® Series!

These handy, accessible books give you all you need to tackle a difficult project, gain a new hobby, comprehend a fascinating topic, prepare for an exam, or even brush up on something you learned back in school but have since forgotten.

You can choose to read an Everything® book from cover to cover or just pick out the information you want from our four useful boxes: e-questions, e-facts, e-alerts, and e-ssentials.

We give you everything you need to know on the subject, but throw in a lot of fun stuff along the way, too.

We now have more than 400 Everything® books in print, spanning such wide-ranging categories as weddings, pregnancy, cooking, music instruction, foreign language, crafts, pets, New Age, and so much more. When you're done reading them all, you can finally say you know Everything®!

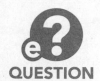
QUESTION
Answers to common questions

FACT
Important snippets of information

ALERT
Urgent warnings

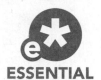
ESSENTIAL
Quick handy tips

PUBLISHER Karen Cooper

MANAGING EDITOR, EVERYTHING® SERIES Lisa Laing

COPY CHIEF Casey Ebert

ASSOCIATE PRODUCTION EDITOR Mary Beth Dolan

ACQUISITIONS EDITOR Lisa Laing

SENIOR DEVELOPMENT EDITOR Laura M. Daly

EVERYTHING® SERIES COVER DESIGNER Erin Alexander

Visit the entire Everything® series at *www.everything.com*

THE
EVERYTHING®
GUIDE TO LIVING GLUTEN-FREE

The ultimate cooking, diet, and lifestyle guide for gluten-free families!

Jeanine Friesen

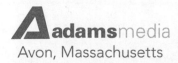

Avon, Massachusetts

To my husband, Chris, and our children, Abigail and Nicholas. Only because of your love and support have I been able to grow my passion for baking, even if it is without gluten.

An Everything® Series Book.
Everything® and everything.com® are registered trademarks of F+W Media, Inc.

Published by Adams Media, a division of F+W Media, Inc. 57 Littlefield Street, Avon, MA 02322. U.S.A.
www.adamsmedia.com

ISBN 10: 1-4405-5184-7
ISBN 13: 978-1-4405-5184-0
eISBN 10: 1-4405-5185-5
eISBN 13: 978-1-4405-5185-7

Printed in the United States of America.

10 9 8 7 6 5 4 3 2

Contains material adapted and abridged from:
The Everything® Food Allergy Cookbook by Linda Larsen, copyright © 2008 by F+W Media, Inc., ISBN 10: 1-59869-560-6, ISBN 13: 978-1-59869-560-1; *The Everything® Vegan Cookbook* by Jolinda Hackett, copyright © 2010 by F+W Media, Inc., ISBN 10: 1-4405-0216-1, ISBN 13: 978-1-4405-0216-3; *The Everything® Gluten-Free Slow Cooker Cookbook* by Carrie Forbes, copyright © 2012 by F+W Media, Inc., ISBN 10: 1-4405-3366-0, ISBN 13: 978-1-4405-3366-2.

This book is available at quantity discounts for bulk purchases. For information, please call 1-800-289-0963.

Contents

Acknowledgments

First and foremost, I need to thank my husband, Christopher, the writer in the family. Chris, without your experience, research, and help, this book would not be what it is. You are supportive, encouraging, and willing to eat anything that I prepare, even when it doesn't turn out the way I expected, and I love you for that.

To my kids, who have grown up with Mom working in the kitchen, and always testing new recipes, thank you for being such fantastic taste-testers. This is not "Mom's book," this is "our book"; everyone in the family contributed to it, and put their energy toward it. I love you guys!

I would also like to say a big thank-you to all the supporters and readers of my blog, "TheBakingBeauties.com." Knowing that I've been able to help you transition to living gluten-free, or that I was able to help you recreate traditions from your pre-gluten-free days, puts a smile on my face every day. Thank you for continuing to fuel my desire to create great gluten-free recipes, so that no one has to go without.

Lastly, a huge thank-you to the people at Adams Media. You believed in me, and that really means a lot. Thank you for the guidance and encouragement during this new adventure.

Top Ten Reasons to Go Gluten-Free

1. You've been diagnosed with celiac disease.

2. You have a wheat allergy or intolerance.

3. Your doctor recommends it.

4. To relieve unexplained gas and bloating.

5. To help alleviate joint pain.

6. You suffer from unexplained infertility or miscarriages.

7. To help reduce the number and intensity of migraine headaches.

8. To try to lessen the effects of ADHD or autism.

9. To support friends, and/or family members, who have to eat gluten-free.

10. Celebrities have been known to drop a few inches while eating gluten-free—why not try it?

Introduction

GLUTEN-FREE. IT'S A PHRASE that's popping up more and more in our society these days. Perhaps you've heard of someone who is eating gluten-free because of digestive problems, or someone else who is doing it to try to alleviate joint pain. Maybe you've heard about a celebrity adopting a gluten-free diet for health and fitness, in hopes of dropping a few dress sizes. Perhaps a local pizza joint is advertising that they are now offering gluten-free pizza crusts, or your favorite bag of chips might have added the words "Gluten-Free" to their packaging. But what does it mean? What is gluten, and why would people need to live a life free of it? And why is the gluten-free diet so prominent in popular culture these days?

Gluten is a previously misunderstood protein that exists in many of the most basic food staples in the standard American diet. What, if anything, has changed in our food that allows a simple whole-wheat sandwich to make someone sick? How can a bowl of cereal for breakfast leave a person doubled over in pain? It turns out that digesting gluten is a problem for many people. The resulting physical symptoms can range in severity from very minor gastrointestinal problems all the way to debilitating pain, migraines, weight loss, infertility, and neurological issues. Other people try to address joint paint, autism, or ADHD with a gluten-free diet. The number of people who eat gluten-free is on the rise, and includes young and old, male and female, discriminating against no one.

The only treatment for the spectrum of gluten-induced disorders is a restrictive gluten-free diet. A gluten-free diet differs from other restrictive diets, like veganism, because a gluten-free diet is, for the most part, not a lifestyle choice. It is the "medicine" needed to get healthy. It's the only prescription, one that lasts a lifetime, for improved health.

What the doctors and dieticians won't tell you about the gluten-free diet is that it is much more than a diet. It is a way of life. When you begin a gluten-free diet, it will change all aspects of your life. Indulging in the doughnuts a coworker brought into work, grabbing a quick snack while heading out the door, and attending a birthday party are normal, everyday events that are affected by a gluten-free diet. You have to stop and think about everything before eating it. And it's not just your food that you need to think about. Medicine, makeup, and craft supplies are all places where gluten can hide as well.

That is where this book comes in. In these pages, you will find 100 great gluten-free recipes to help you get started on your gluten-free diet, as well as information that will help you gain insight into how to live a full life totally free of gluten. You will find tips on setting up your gluten-free kitchen, advice on how to travel and still maintain a gluten-free diet, and suggestions on how to help a child cope with a gluten-free life.

But a gluten-free life isn't all about loss and restrictions. It is also about variety and abundance and finding new ways to enjoy your life. Just because your diet cannot contain gluten doesn't mean it has to be devoid of flavor, excitement, or variety. With some forethought and planning, you can still entertain, you can still go out, and you can still indulge in many of your favorite traditional foods. This book will help you embrace and live your gluten-free life to the fullest and help you reap the reward of long-term health through living gluten-free.

CHAPTER 1

Gluten 101

When you think of a gluten-free life, do you imagine a dinner of rice cakes, carrot sticks, and water? A lifetime without juicy burgers, plates of pasta, and chocolate cake? Thankfully, in reality, the gluten-free life is nothing like that. Embracing and enjoying a gluten-free life is possible and it doesn't have to be bland and boring. But getting there—eliminating those misconceptions and realizing that you are, in fact, in for exciting new lifestyle and culinary experiences—requires some knowledge and planning. This chapter is designed to explain what gluten is, where it can be found, and how it got there. Only by understanding these subjects will it be possible to live free of gluten.

What Is Gluten?

You've probably heard of gluten. Maybe it was from a high school home economics teacher explaining how bread gets its structure and texture. Or maybe it was on the cooking show you watched the other day, where the host made a sourdough bread recipe and explained how important it was to knead the dough in order for the dough to become elastic. Or maybe a doctor has recently presented a diagnosis of celiac disease and informed you that you will need to avoid foods containing gluten. Most people, if they've spent any amount of time preparing food, are familiar with the term. But what *is* gluten?

How Gluten Forms

That home economics teacher and the cooking show host are both right: Gluten is what allows flour to be made into bread loaves, rolls, and cakes. Gluten is actually the combination of two microscopic proteins, *glutenin* and *gliadin*, which occur naturally in many cereal grains, including wheat, barley, and rye. These two proteins exist independently and randomly within the whole head of the grain, and within the grain's flour, once it has been milled. They are not soluble in water and are what gives wheat dough its elastic texture.

Wheat kernels are covered by a fibrous shell of bran, making up approximately 14 percent of its total weight. Inside the bran, a white, nutrient-rich substance, known as the endosperm, accounts for approximately 83 percent of the kernel's weight. The germ, the embryo or "sprouting" part of the seed, makes up only about 2.5 percent of the kernel's weight. All three parts contain the proteins that make gluten.

The large, starchy endosperm provides the food necessary during seed germination. Moisture absorbed by the grain activates enzymes, which begin to break the starches and proteins (*glutenin* and *gliadin*) down and supply the fledgling plant with the molecular nourishment necessary to break through the soil and reach for the sky. As the plant grows, the roots begin to absorb the nutrients needed to fuel plant growth and fruit (seed) development. The daughter seeds contain the same starchy, protein-rich endosperm as the mother seed. Once harvested and ground, the endosperm becomes the white part of baking flour. Since sprouting begins to break down the gluten-forming proteins, sprouted seeds contain less gluten, but sprouting does not eliminate the gluten content entirely.

Adding water to cereal grain flour begins a chemical reaction in which the two proteins start to align and combine. Kneading the flour/water mixture speeds the chemical reactions that are transforming what were two independent proteins into the new protein known as gluten. The longer the dough is mixed, the more developed and aligned the gluten protein becomes.

As the gluten is formed, it develops physical properties that are similar to the surface of a rubber balloon. These properties allow dough mixtures to stretch and expand as the leavening agent (usually yeast) produces carbon dioxide bubbles in a separate chemical reaction.

As the carbon dioxide bubbles form, the gluten forms pockets around them, giving bread and other baked goods their final structure and texture. The baking process stops the chemical reactions by drying out the dough and solidifying the gluten protein strands in their final state. It is possible to see strands of gluten when dough is well kneaded by simply stretching the dough as thin as possible without tearing. Once the dough is thin enough that it becomes translucent, holding it up to a light produces a "baker's window" where long strands of developed gluten will show up as dark lines in the dough.

Varying Types of Gluten

By breeding different varieties of grain, different flours with different amounts of gluten-forming proteins have been developed. Bakers can select flour varieties that will produce the best-baked product:

- **Higher-gluten-content flours** are used for breads that need to be tough and durable, able to hold up a pile of toppings without crumbling into dust.
- **Lower-gluten-content flours** are used for cakes and pastries that still require strength and structure but also require delicacy.

In both cases, gluten is the mesh of molecules that provides that support.

The Natural History of Wheat

Around 10,000 years ago, humans began to grow and process cereal grains. This early agricultural production marked the human transition from nomadic hunter-gatherers to semi-permanent agricultural societies, eventually leading ancient people to become permanent community dwellers. Agrarian society soon gave rise to early civilization, and cereal grains continued to be important crops in the global food supply. As civilization has advanced and changed, it has, in turn, changed the grains that were so instrumental in its early formation.

Early Wheat Production

The domestication of modern wheat started in the fertile crescent of the ancient Near East. The ancestors of modern wheat include a pair of wild grasses known as einkorn (*Triticum monococcum*) and emmer (*Triticum dicoccum*). As early farmers grew these two varieties, they selected seeds from the best plants to use in later growing seasons. Early domestication focused on producing varieties that made plants more productive and easier to harvest.

Einkorn

Early agricultural efforts were labor intensive and the grains themselves did little to help. As plants—essentially, wild-growing grasses—these grains had no consideration for human need. Their purpose was to grow and disperse their seeds as widely as possible, ensuring that a new generation would grow the following year. To achieve this, these plants naturally germinated when conditions were right for the seeds. The rachis, the thin connecting spine that holds the seedpods, was brittle and easily shattered, ensuring dispersal at the time of ripening. Early cereals also had hulled grains, a tough casing around the seed to keep it protected, and a small seed. These traits made it difficult to grow and process an entire crop in a uniform and efficient manner.

FACT

In a study published in a November 1997 issue of *Science* magazine, researchers reported that they had discovered the site of the domestication of einkorn wheat. Using DNA fingerprinting, the researchers determined that a wild group of *Triticum monococcum boeoticum* from the Karacadağ Mountains in southeastern Turkey are the "likely" progenitors of cultivated einkorn. Evidence from nearby archaeological excavations supported the DNA findings.

Domestication efforts, whether by earlier experience, intuition, or simply luck, sought to combat these agricultural problems by breeding varieties that resisted shattering, germinated more uniformly, and were easier to hull during threshing. Domestication also sought to favor larger seeds.

Emmer

Emmer wheat has a similar story, with wild varieties occurring naturally around the Fertile Crescent before giving rise to domesticated varieties. Emmer production was more widespread than einkorn, and emmer has the distinguished honor of being the great-grandfather of the modern varieties of bread and durum wheat.

Hybridization

From the Fertile Crescent and the ancient Near East, domesticated varieties began to spread throughout the Middle East into parts of Asia, Africa, and Europe. After these early domestications, and possibly due to the migration of wheat to other areas, hybridization with other species began to occur, forming new varieties with desirable traits. Human-directed plant breeding has continued throughout history until the emergence of modern varieties in the 1970s. Today, thanks to these efforts, every month of the year a crop of wheat can be harvested somewhere in the world.

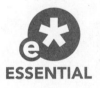

ESSENTIAL

Domestication and trait selection in agriculture is not unique to wheat. Other plants have undergone the same treatment. Just think of the variety of apples available in a modern grocery store or the types of tomatoes available for use on sandwiches, in salads, or for making sauces. It's important to have variety because, even though a Roma tomato will work in a sandwich, a juicy round beefsteak or hothouse works much better.

Emmer and einkorn wheat are still grown today, primarily around the Mediterranean. Now considered relict crops or ancient grains, they grow well in marginal land. Even in poor soils, the grain produced is high in protein. Einkorn protein levels are estimated to be 12–13.5 percent higher than barley, while estimates for emmer place their protein levels at 5–35 percent higher than oats or barley.

The Green Revolution

Ancient domestication efforts were centered on producing a crop more suitable for ancient farming and threshing techniques. In the last hundred years or so, agronomists have turned their attention to other matters. After World War II, worldwide food shortages threatened many Third-World nations.

One of the most influential advances in the breeding of modern wheat occurred in the early twentieth century, when the "reduced height gene" was introduced into crop populations around the world. The reduced height gene, called Rht8 (along with another gene identified as Ppd-D1), decreased the height of wheat by four inches and improved the onset of flowering by eight days. All this change and improvement did have a positive effect. Wheat production around the world began to increase, and along with it, the food security in developing nations. This "green revolution" was achieved, not by increasing the area of cultivated land, but by increasing the productivity of the plants being grown. Some estimates put the increase at 250 percent higher yields.

FACT

The global trade for wheat is larger than all other crops combined. It is grown on more than 240 million hectares of land, worldwide, which is larger than for any other crop. Global wheat consumption reached about 550 million tonnes per year in 1990 with recent years approaching 700 million tonnes. Wheat is a primary source for vitamins, minerals, and dietary fiber for much of the world's population. Some estimates place wheat's contribution to the daily intake of iron at 44 percent and zinc at 25 percent in developed countries.

As good as this all sounds, the green revolution hasn't come without impacts in other areas. Modern commercial farming requires large amounts of fertilizer, water use, and increased reliance on pesticides to protect the crops. The commercialization of wheat production also led to an increase in the mechanization of planting and harvesting, which led to the need for more fuel and increased costs for farmers. Ecologically, soil quality has declined as intensive farming operations grow multiple crops during the same year. Water quality has also suffered from the introduction and overuse of pesticides into the environment.

But perhaps the most concerning is the reduction in genetic diversity. Modern wheat varieties are characterized by their uniformity. According to the Food and Agriculture Organization of the United Nations, this monoculture within agriculture is the main cause of the loss of genetic diversity, which has negative implications on its nutritional qualities. Indeed, the ancient varieties of grain all show a large amount of variation in size and shape, but the modern "elite" varieties that have been derived from these ancestors are all similar in size and shape. Line them up side by side and the ancient grains vary in length, width, and shape. Their modern counterparts, however, all have a uniform plumpness to them and are roughly equal in length.

The Green Revolution's Effect on Nutritional Content

Protein content (*gliadin* and *glutenin*) is largely dependent on several factors. Crop selection and breeding has played a role in producing higher-protein varieties, but environmental factors like timing and amount of precipitation, temperature, or heat during the growing season—and especially the nitrogen content of the soil—will affect the protein content of wheat. Since the agricultural techniques developed during the green revolution rely on an increased application of nitrogen-based fertilizer, gluten and protein content in modern wheat varieties are much higher. Some studies have been conducted demonstrating that the application of nitrogen to wheat, at the correct time during its growing season, can increase the gluten content of the grains twofold.

As for other nutrients important to humans, in 2006, plant researchers with the U.S. Department of Agriculture published the results of a study that examined the concentration of nutrients essential to humans, specifically of iron, zinc, copper, and selenium. The researchers studied fourteen varieties of hard red winter wheat that were developed between 1874 and 1995. The studies found that as newer wheat varieties were developed into higher-yielding crops, the nutrient content, including that of iron, zinc, and selenium, decreased.

One Doctor's Take on the Green Revolution's Effect on Wheat

With its importance and prevalence in the human diet, knowing how wheat affects human health seems very important. Recently, wheat has come under increased scrutiny due to low-carbohydrate diets and an increase in celiac and gluten allergy diagnoses. In addition, some people suffering from other seemingly unrelated disorders like autism, ADHD, and schizophrenia have benefited from removing wheat from their diet, further fueling the suspicion about wheat's harmful effects.

Dr. William Davis, MD, a preventive cardiologist from Milwaukee, Wisconsin, has recognized these effects and has begun a campaign against wheat's use in commercial food products. His research has led him to conclude that modern wheat is different from the wheat that was available in the early 1900s, very different from the wheat varieties available in the mid-1800s, and completely different from what helped establish ancient civilizations in the distant past. His online writings draw a conclusion between green revolution agriculture and this dramatic change in wheat.

"Something happened to wheat in the 1970s during the efforts to generate a high-yield strain that required less fertilizer to make a 24-inch, rather than a 48-inch, stalk," Dr. Davis writes in one post on his website, *www .wheatbellyblog.com*. That "something" goes way beyond the physical traits of the plant. Dr. Davis is convinced that modern wheat varieties are addictive, even going so far as to call them an "opiate."

"Wheat is addictive in the sense that it comes to dominate thoughts and behaviours," Davis writes. "Wheat is addictive in the sense that, if you don't have any for several hours, you start to get nervous, foggy, tremulous, and start desperately seeking out another 'hit' of crackers, bagels, or bread."

Dr. Davis became convinced that wheat was contributing to the ill health of his patients when they came to him as diabetic or prediabetic. His advice was simple: Eliminate wheat from your diet.

"Foods made of wheat flour raise blood sugar higher than nearly all other foods," he says. "More than table sugar, more than a Snickers bar."

Not only did eliminating wheat from their diet help with regulating their blood sugar, his patients also began noticing weight loss and relief from a variety of other symptoms including relief from arthritis, asthma, and irritable bowel syndrome, and they enjoyed more stable moods and better sleep.

Why Is Gluten in Food?

Gluten exists in food products because cereal grains like wheat, barley, and rye are important, legitimate ingredients in many different types of foods. You can't have breaded chicken without breading, can you? A Caesar salad could be made without croutons, but then it wouldn't be a Caesar salad, would it? And what makes a Danish pastry a pastry? Isn't it the delicate dough that supports the fruit filling and the drizzle of sweet icing? These examples are all understandable, and the fact that those foods include gluten shouldn't come as a surprise. But the fact is that, historically, gluten has also existed in food products for less obvious reasons.

Chocolate History

Going back to the mid-1800s, gluten was an important part of chocolate manufacturing. In fact, people seemed to believe that both chocolate and the gluten added to it provided positive health benefits and could help people grow. One patent specification from England in 1853, published in *Specifications Relating to Cooking, Bread-Making, and the Preparation of Confectionery,* states that, "Chocolate and vermicelli may be made with gluten." Later in the passage, the broad strokes of the recipe are given. "Gluten chocolate," it says, is "composed of about two parts of cocoa and one part of gluten bread, reduced to an impalpable powder." Several variations on the same recipe followed, some adding sugar, others adding "muriatic acid," but all involving some form of gluten, either as "pulverized" bread or "pure gluten flour."

The *New American Cyclopædia: A Popular Dictionary of General Knowledge,* from 1867, explains that "starch, gum, gluten and the large proportions of fat give cocoa the variety of nutritive quantities contained in milk, and like this [*sic*] it contains every ingredient necessary to the growth and sustenance of the body."

This notion of nutritive benefit can also be found in an advertisement from the same era for Cadbury's Cocoa Essence. The ad extols the health benefits of a large breakfast cup of hot cocoa by quoting a study published in *The Lancet* in 1867, which refers to the added gluten as "stimulating" and "flesh-forming."

Coffee and Tea History

Coffee and tea also have an interesting historical connection to wheat. In 1718, the King of England, George I, enacted a law that prevented coffee dealers from adding impurities to coffee in an effort to increase its bulk and their own profits. The law was designed to preserve the health of his subjects and protect honest and fair dealers in the commodity from the use of contaminants like grease and butter. Later in 1803, King George III expanded on the law to prevent the use of "scorched, or roasted peas, beans, or other grains, or vegetable substance" in adulterating coffee. While it's more difficult to find examples of how wheat might have been used to adulterate tea, it can't be entirely dismissed. As the popularity of tea rose in England, a shadow industry was fraudulently putting adulterated products on the market. Eventually tea laws, similar in intent to the coffee laws, were passed to prevent the adulteration of tea.

Chocolate, Coffee, and Tea Today

Gluten is rarely used as an ingredient in modern chocolate production anymore; however, gluten may still appear in trace amounts through the use of other ingredients. "Barley malt syrup" and "wheat glucose syrup" are still common additives. So is wheat starch, which is used to dust chocolate molds to make it easier to remove the finished chocolate. Even though the chocolate may have been made without any gluten-containing ingredients, the entire product, covered in wheat starch, technically contains gluten.

QUESTION

How can I be sure the coffee and chocolate I buy is gluten-free?
Most chocolate and coffee companies will tell you directly if their products are gluten-free. Some readily answer these questions on their websites. Check the manufacturer's "Frequently Asked Questions" page and if you can't find the answer there, make the question more frequent by asking it yourself.

Today, coffee is rarely adulterated with gluten-containing products. The King of England outlawed it centuries ago, after all. Extra care should be taken with herbal teas, as some brands and flavors include roasted barley.

Flavored chocolate and coffee beverages, and those with flavored coffee whiteners, should also be watched carefully, as these products often use sweeteners that have been derived from gluten-producing grains.

Where Is Gluten Found?

Regardless of how large a gluten molecule strand may become during the baking process, gluten will always remain microscopic. This can make gluten difficult to detect. Gluten can be found in obvious places like breads and other baked goods—crackers, cookies, and pastries. But it can also be found in less obvious places. Understanding where gluten is found, in large quantities, is the first step in being able to predict where it might appear in small quantities.

Gluten shows up in many foods because wheat is still being used everywhere in commercial food production. Everything from licorice to canned soup may contain wheat flour and, for the celiac or gluten intolerant, every commercial food product should be suspect. Some other common items that may contain gluten include:

- Gravy and bouillon cubes
- Ice cream
- Pie fillings
- Ketchup
- Salad dressing
- Bottled sauces
- Candy bars
- As a thickening or binding agent in soups and sauces
- As an anti-caking ingredient in seasoning mixes
- Meat products containing binders or fillers

There are two products that account for much of the gluten contamination in commercial foods like these: barley malt syrup and good ol' wheat gluten.

Wheat Gluten

There is an entire industry whose sole purpose is to process wheat into a "free-flowing powder of high protein content and bland taste" so its "exceptional functionality" may be used by "many industries by imparting a variety of benefits." That's according to the International Wheat Gluten Association (IWGA). The IWGA is made up of member companies who process wheat gluten and supply it as an ingredient to various industries, including commercial food and cosmetic companies.

Wheat gluten is extracted from wheat by a variety of processes, some of which go back to 1835. Most of the processes are similar and consist of adding water to raw wheat flour, forming dough. Once the dough is fully formed and hydrated, more water is added to begin separating the gluten from the starch. A screening process further separates the wet gluten from the starch.

FACT

The Martin process for gluten extraction was developed in 1835 in Paris. Its major drawback was excessive water waste. The Batter process was invented in 1944, and more recently a Dutch company has developed a hydrocyclone process that recycles wash water, almost eliminating the problem of water waste and making it the most popular method of gluten extraction. Other processes are named after the companies that developed them and include Pillsbury Hydromilling, Alfa-Laval/Raisio, Modified "Fesca," Alkali, and Far-Mar-Co.

Regardless of the process, the finished product has proven to be a very versatile component in many consumer products. Wheat gluten is so functional and unique, and according to the IWGA website, "so persistent in structural integrity," even after being processed or cooked that, "it appears to have no functional competitor."

So what is all this wheat gluten used for? The IWGA lists several industries:

- Aquaculture (fish food)
- Breading, batters, coatings, and flavors
- Breakfast cereals
- Cheese substitutes
- Meat, fish, poultry, and surimi (imitation crab meat)-based products
- Natural biopolymers such as cellophane and other plastics

- Pet foods
- Baked goods

In the United States, the Food and Drug Administration regulates gluten and has affirmed it as "Generally Recognized as Safe" for use for a variety of purposes, including as a nutrient supplement, processing aid, stabilizer and thickener, finishing and texturing agent, and dough strengthener. With this approval and all the potential uses, it's easy to see how gluten can be found in so many "everyday" products. Gluten is also used in other countries for producing monosodium glutamate seasoning and gluten hydrolysate, which is often incorporated into soy sauce as an extender.

The American Institute of Baking's (AIB) research department issued a Technical Bulletin in 1994 that documented the use of wheat gluten in food and nonfood systems. The bulletin explains that:

- Gluten has "meat-like" characteristics and binding properties that make its use widespread. It is used to produce loaves of meat with good slice-ability and in "simulated" meat products that can be blended with real meat to produce sausages and hamburger patties.
- Other food uses include edible and odor-free films and coatings used to wrap or encase cheese, sandwiches, and hors d'oeuvres, and as moisture barriers for candy.
- Wheat gluten and its derivatives can be used in adhesives, cigarette filters, and pharmaceutical tablets.
- Wheat gluten has also been used as a component in chewing gums to "make it more hygienic, palatable, nutritional and readily digestible, if accidentally swallowed."

Barley Malt Syrup

Barley malt syrup is an ever-present ingredient that is easily overlooked by those seeking to avoid gluten-containing ingredients. It's barley, after all, not wheat. But barley is one of the gluten-containing cereal crops, and products derived from it are guilty by association.

Barley malt syrup, sometimes simply called malt syrup, is a sweetener made from malted barley. The process is simple; barley is washed and placed in a tank to soak until the grains have absorbed enough moisture.

They are then turned out onto a sprouting bed, where the controlled heat and moisture allow them to sprout. Once sprouted, the barley is rapidly dried in kilns to stop the germination but preserve the enzymes activated during the sprouting stage. The dried, sprouted barley is then crushed or mashed with more moisture and the resulting liquids are strained and evaporated to produce the desired viscosity while the solids are used as high-quality animal feed.

While it might not be as sweet as refined white sugar—most estimates put malt syrup at about half the sweetness—its distinct malted flavor has made it desirable as an ingredient in many products, like chocolate and cereal.

Malted barley also adds bulk and binding to products; acts as a natural humectant (a substance that helps a product retain water); and enhances browning, fermentation, body, and viscosity. Typical products that contain malt syrup include:

- Malted milk balls
- Cough drops
- Candies
- Energy bars
- Popcorn
- Baby foods
- Soy milk
- Yogurt
- Brown sugar
- Table syrup
- Peanut butter

Again, since barley is not technically wheat, people with gluten sensitivities might be tempted to try to eat barley products like malt syrup. Research on this topic is ongoing. Dr. Donald D. Kasarda, PhD, is a former research chemist with the USDA. He says in a post on the USDA website that it is difficult to quantify the toxicity of any grain type and that it is possible that barley is less toxic than wheat for those with gluten sensitivities. He also says that since barley malt is produced from the sprouted grain, most of the gluten-forming proteins that the seedling uses for food in the early stages of development have been broken down, further reducing the toxicity.

He never says that barley or barley malt syrup isn't toxic to those with gluten sensitivities, but he does repeatedly state that more research is needed in this area. The bottom line is: if it has the potential to cause harm to your system, it's probably not worth eating.

Cross-Contamination

Crumbs from bread, crackers, cookies, and pastries can appear anywhere these products are handled. If these products find their way into other food items as ingredients (a process known as cross-contamination), even in small amounts, they can cause unhealthy reactions in people with gluten sensitivities.

ALERT

Even trace amounts of gluten can cause severe reactions in people with celiac disease. A study conducted in 2004 attempted to find a safe threshold for gluten contamination. While the researchers acknowledged that a gluten-free diet should be as strict as possible, their study concluded that the acceptable threshold for gluten contamination in food products is 100 parts per million (PPM). Food that is manufactured and certified "gluten-free" measured in at 20 PPM or lower. A slice of regular white bread contains approximately 350 times more gluten than is safe for a person with celiac disease to consume.

Cross-contamination can turn an ordinary kitchen into a toxic waste depot for people with celiac disease. Just think of what's lying at the bottom of a toaster. Even if you put a slice of gluten-free bread in that toaster, it's likely going to come into contact with gluten-filled bread crumbs. Or, consider Uncle Bob at Thanksgiving. He has the annoying habit of dragging the gravy ladle *through* the stuffing on his plate before returning it to the buffet's gravy bowl. Unbeknownst to Uncle Bob, he has just contaminated the gravy with gluten.

Cross-contamination can also occur from the manufacturing equipment used in the commercial food processing industry. Much like peanut residue on improperly cleaned equipment can pose a health risk to those suffering from peanut allergies, trace amounts of gluten can be incorporated into food and pose a health risk to celiac sufferers and gluten-intolerant people. This problem can extend all the way back through the manufacturing chain to the farmer's field, where the grain was first grown. For example, oats don't contain gluten, but if they are grown on the same field that produced a crop of wheat the previous year, at harvest time, the threshing machines won't be able to tell the difference and some amount of wheat will be mixed in with the oats. Grain hauling, handling, storage, and processing equipment can all be early sources of gluten contact and contamination.

Restaurants and commercial kitchens suffer from the same problem. Though many do their best, the possibility of allergen cross-contamination can never be fully eliminated. Deep fryers are a hot spot for gluten contamination if the same oil used for cooking French fries is also used for cooking breaded chicken or fish.

Beverages

Don't forget about your favorite beverages. Beer is made from wheat, rye, and barley and contains gluten. There is some anecdotal evidence that the distillation process used to make beer eliminates the gluten, but studies have shown that even beer labeled "low gluten" contains dangerously high levels for people with gluten sensitivities.

QUESTION

Does wine contain gluten?
Although not yet a common fining agent in the winemaking process, gluten's use has been gaining popularity. Scientists began studying its suitability several years ago, when concerns about mad cow disease were raised over gelatin, the industry's preferred fining agent. Pea protein, milk protein, egg whites, and fish glue have all been used for wine fining. Bentonite clay can also be used and is both gluten-free and vegan.

Wine, on the other hand, is made from a naturally gluten-free fruit, so you'd assume that it's gluten-free, right? Wrong. Grapes alone are perfectly safe to eat fresh, dried, juiced, or fermented. However, some wine is aged in wood barrels that have been sealed with flour-based sealants, and gluten may be used as a clarifying agent in the "fining" process.

CHAPTER 2

Celiac Disease

When you first heard the phrase "celiac disease," you probably had a lot of questions: What is it? If you have it, how did you get it? Who else is affected? The fact is, before you can fight your "enemy," you have to understand it. While gluten may be your enemy, understanding your enemy's tactics in your body is key to forming a counterattack strategy. Celiac disease has a long history, but much of the understanding has come from very recent advancements in research. This new understanding has led to better and more accurate diagnostic tests, and may one day lead to better therapeutic options for treatment.

Early Researchers

What we now know commonly as celiac disease has been described in medical literature as far back as the first century A.D.

Aretaeus of Cappadocia

A Greek physician named Aretaeus of Cappadocia described a condition where the stomach was "irretentive of food" and where "nothing ascends into the body" of the afflicted person. Aretaeus, with his apt observations, named this condition *koiliakos,* after the Greek word for abdomen: "*koelia.*" Aretaeus was a careful observer and remarkably advanced clinician for his time. He vividly recorded his clinical descriptions in eight volumes of writings.

Aretaeus somehow understood that properly digested food was integrated into the body, somewhere in the belly organs. He was also careful to note that the condition he was describing was chronic and recurring, not transient and only lasting a day or two. His observations state that people affected produced foul-smelling, discolored, unformed "digestive product" or "flatulent product." He also noted severe, intermittent abdominal pain; starvation; patients who were pallid and feeble, having no energy to perform any of the usual functions; and dehydration.

FACT

Aretaeus of Cappadocia is considered one of the greatest physicians of Greco-Roman antiquity. He is believed to have been trained in Alexandria and practiced in Rome. He is credited with being the first physician to distinguish between transmission of a disease through contact with a contagion and at a distance by infection. In addition to clearly documenting the symptoms of celiac disease, Aretaeus's writings also provided early descriptions of asthma, pneumonia, cerebral apoplexy (stroke), tetanus, hysteria, epilepsy, gout, diphtheria, and diabetes.

Aretaeus believed digestion was the result of a natural heat, dwelling within the body. He surmised that the symptoms he observed were caused by a chilling of that heat. Remarkably, he prescribed treatment that included rest and fasting—a drastic modification in the diet—to relieve the stress on the patients' bowels. Aretaeus only recorded his observations of the disease in adult patients. He thought the disease to affect mainly the elderly and women and missed its prevalence in children.

It took almost 1,800 years before anyone would significantly follow up on Aretaeus's work. In the late 1800s and early 1900s, a string of physicians, working with children, would grow the base of available information on celiac disease, laying the foundation for a modern understanding of the disease.

Samuel Gee

Samuel Jones Gee was born in London in 1839. His career as a physician was marked by a thriving practice, prestigious appointments, and a bibliography of important medical publications. In 1888, borrowing a title from Aretaeus, and using the British spelling, he wrote an account of what he called "the Coeliac Affection." Published in the *St. Bartholomew's Hospital Reports*, the account reflected the observations he had made a year earlier, while giving a lecture at the Hospital for Sick Children in London. He described the condition as: "a kind of chronic indigestion which is met with in persons of all ages, yet is especially apt to affect children between one and five years old."

ESSENTIAL

In 2010, in honor of Samuel Gee's contribution to the modern understanding of celiac disease, the U.S. Senate declared Gee's birthday, September 13, as National Celiac Awareness Day. Accordingly, the Senate resolution called for all people of the United States to "become more informed and aware of Celiac Disease" and observe "appropriate ceremonies and activities" to mark the occasion.

Gee realized that the problem was probably diet-related and even stated that the only means of curing a patient would be through a modified diet. But despite having performed more than 600 necropsies, Gee failed to observe the physical effects of celiac disease on the intestines. He did, however, describe in vivid detail the nature of the feces of affected patients as "being loose, not formed, but not watery; more bulky than the food taken would seem to account for; pale in color, as if devoid of bile; yeasty, frothy, an appearance probably due to fermentation; stinking, stench often very great, the food having undergone putrefaction rather than concoction."

Shortly before Gee's death, another physician was observing the effect celiac disease was having on children. While his contribution to our modern understanding of the disease isn't as large as Gee's, Christian Herter's work, in its own way, added to the modern understanding of the condition.

Christian Archibald Herter

Christian Archibald Herter was an American contemporary of Samuel Gee's. Born in 1865, he died a year earlier than Gee in 1910 at the age of 45. Despite his short life, Herter was a notable man of medical science. He believed in the use of pure research and the incorporation of other branches of science—chemistry, physics, and sociology—in determining the cause of disease. His influence on modern understandings of disease was vast. He was the cofounder and first editor of the *Journal of Biological Chemistry* and set up two lectureships, one in New York and one in Baltimore, to further the medical knowledge of his colleagues.

FACT

Christian Herter's father, an artist and interior decorator/architect, chose medicine for his son's career. His father enrolled Herter in medical school when the boy was fifteen years old and he received his MD only three years later. Herter believed so strongly in the use of research in the pursuit of understanding diseases, that he established a private laboratory on the top floor of his home. He used his father's wealth to sustain the laboratory and the medical journal he co-founded.

Herter's interest in science and chemistry led to detailed studies on intestinal micro-organisms. In his study of celiac disease, which he termed "Intestinal Infatilism," Herter noted two major items. Like Gee, he noticed that afflicted children failed to thrive, that their growth was stunted by the condition. And perhaps more importantly, Herter discovered that a diet of fat was better tolerated than a diet rich in carbohydrates—foreshadowing later discoveries about gluten.

Willem Karel Dicke

Willem Karel Dicke, born in 1905, was another pioneering researcher in celiac disease and its treatment. He would have just been entering his elementary education in his native Netherlands around the time Gee and Herter died.

When Dicke began practicing medicine, celiac disease was commonly referred to as "Gee-Herter" disease, and the two main treatments were rest and an altered diet. Another outstanding man of medical science, Dicke ascended to the position of medical director of the Juliana Children's Hospital in The Hague at the age of thirty-one. Twelve years earlier, Sidney Haas had published a study describing his treatment of celiac disease with a banana diet. His study was dramatic, eight patients treated with the banana diet were clinically cured and two who had maintained their normal diet actually died. At a conference in 1932, Dicke heard a report about a patient relapsing into diarrhea after resuming the consumption of bread. According to Dicke's wife, he began experimenting with a wheat-free diet shortly thereafter, between 1934 and 1936. His first report of his tests with wheat-free diets was published in 1941.

Then came World War II, and in its aftermath, a "Winter of Starvation" from 1944 to 1955. During that time, food in general—and bread in particular—was scarce. Dicke was further convinced that removing wheat from his patients' diet was essential for improving their condition. Since Willem Karel Dicke was the first to draw a connection between wheat and celiac disease, he is credited as being the pioneer of the gluten-free diet.

More Recent Developments in Celiac Research

Despite these early researchers' best efforts, they were able to determine little more than a very basic outline of celiac disease. But they laid the groundwork for a large number of modern researchers who have carried on their work. There are many scientists and medical facilities continuing to study celiac disease, but some of the most important current research is being conducted by the Center for Celiac Research at the University of Maryland, School of Medicine. Dr. Alessio Fasano is the director and it was his group that, in 2003, published the results of a study showing that 1 in 133 people in the United States were affected by celiac disease.

ESSENTIAL

Dr. Fasano's 2003 study was the result of the largest hunt for people with celiac disease in North America. The study involved more than 13,000 people. Celiac disease had long been considered rare, but Dr. Fasano's study showed that it was much more common, approximately 100 times more common in North America, than previously thought. Since then, similar studies have been done on every other continent leading to similar findings in many countries.

What Exactly Is Celiac Disease?

Dr. Fasano, in his 2003 study of the frequency of celiac disease, defined the disorder as follows: "Celiac disease is an immune-mediated enteropathic condition triggered in genetically susceptible individuals by the ingestion of gluten."

More commonly, the popular medical media refers to celiac disease as an autoimmune disorder that damages the small intestine, and, generally, causes flu-like symptoms after gluten has been ingested. What is "immune-mediation" or "autoimmunity"? It's a unique situation where the body's immune system begins to treat itself as an invading pathogen—the body attacks itself instead of attacking the material that's causing the immune response.

Gluten Hates Your Guts

It may seem childish to refer to the stomach, intestines, and associated organs as "guts," but that's exactly what scientists do. The gastrointestinal (GI) tract is often referred to in scientific literature as the gut, and one of the most prestigious scientific journals publishing research into its disorders is simply referred to as *Gut*.

What researchers like Dr. Fasano and others have realized is that gluten has long had a poor relationship with our guts, a history going back to the very advent of agriculture. They have been discovering that the way gluten influences the body and causes problems stems from a variety of factors—a perfect storm of conditions—that meet in the guts of susceptible people to trigger the symptoms.

ALERT

A team of researchers from Sweden and South Africa estimate that 42,000 children, mainly from Africa and Asia, die from celiac disease each year. Children in these regions suffer in poorer settings where other diarrheal diseases are common and lack of information can prevent a proper diagnosis. The researchers admit the study is based on estimates and assumptions due to a lack of reliable data, but they hope to raise awareness so that, in addition to preventing needless deaths, more reliable data can be collected.

The Inner Workings of the Gut

For all their otherwise vulgar functions, the human intestines are remarkably intricate organs. Intestines are complex biochemical machines with an architecture designed to simultaneously process a variety of functions that help keep humans healthy. Much of the work happens at a molecular level, but basically, in a healthy individual, after passing through the stomach, food particles enter the small intestine, where they are broken down into component nutrients and absorbed into the bloodstream for use in the body.

The small intestine is a tube of layered tissues that does the work of digesting food and absorbing nutrients. It is also the battleground where the immune system first confronts foreign particles that the body determines to be harmful. The inner layer of the intestine is made up of long rows of enterocytes. Enterocytes are shaped, roughly, like a hand. Place a lot of hands next to each other and you have good idea what the inner lining of an intestine looks like. The fingers, projecting into the tube of the intestine, represent the villi. Under the enterocyte, layers of tissue, containing immune system cells, separate the intestine from the bloodstream. Enterocytes are joined to each other in a molecular bond approximately at the point where the thumbs are. This bond is known simply as a "tight junction."

The villi are responsible for breaking down food particles and incorporating the nutrients into the bloodstream. Under normal circumstances, the food particles are admitted through the enterocyte's structure. Imagine the food being absorbed through the fingers, moving through the palms and passing through the wrist joints to eventually get into the bloodstream. Cellular probes within the intestine continuously interrogate the incoming material to determine if a particle is a "good guy," like food, or an "enemy," like harmful bacteria or a virus. All the material is tagged, and depending on what the molecules determine, the intestines will absorb or combat the particle as necessary. If the intestines decide to combat the particle, immune system cells from the layers under the enterocytes will pass through the enterocytes—back up through the palm—and enter the intestine.

The Effects of Gluten in a Person with Celiac Disease

Gluten disrupts these normal processes in several ways in those with celiac disease. First, gluten is a protein that the body naturally finds difficult to digest. Once it gets into the lower intestine, it presents itself as a foreign body that causes the enterocytes to release a chemical that loosens the tight molecular junctions between cells. Recall that the tight junctions are formed between the enterocytes, still using the hand analogy, where the thumbs would meet when placing the hands beside each other. These tight junctions aren't intended to be opened under normal circumstances. But opening them creates what Dr. Fasano refers to as a "leaky gut" and allows the gluten particles to launch a second attack.

Gluten molecules pass through these junctions and penetrate directly to the layer of immune cells under the enterocytes. That's where the real damage begins, as the enterocytes release a chemical, which marshals the immune system response. Unfortunately, the communication in the ranks breaks down, causing a mutiny. The immune system cells begin to rebel against the very body they are supposed to be protecting. They end up attacking and damaging the enterocytes. Damaged enterocytes can't perform their normal function of breaking down and absorbing nutrients and the body responds with a wide spectrum of disorders or symptoms.

Signs and Symptoms

Celiac disease has a classical set of symptoms. Aretaeus observed that his patients' stomachs were "irretentive of food"—a polite way of saying they suffered from diarrhea. Indeed, being an affliction of the intestines, one of the main, often chronic symptoms associated with celiac disease is diarrhea. Along with diarrhea, celiac patients often experience intestinal bloating and cramps.

Other symptoms that may be less obviously associated with celiac disease can include irritability and weight loss. With the nutrient uptake system under attack, much-needed nutrients entering the intestines never get absorbed before being passed from the body. Nutrient deficiencies like anemia are commonly related to celiac disease. Failure to incorporate nutrients from the food supply can also lead to fatigue.

Any combination of the following symptoms can occur in a person who has celiac disease. The severity of the symptoms may also vary. Unfortunately, many of these symptoms mimic other conditions, such as irritable bowel syndrome, lactose intolerance, or diverticulosis. The following symptoms may occur alone, or in combination with others:

- Diarrhea
- Anemia
- Fatigue
- Joint pain
- Canker sores
- Depression
- Irritability
- Infertility
- Constipation
- Weight loss
- Vitamin deficiency

Children with celiac disease may display any of these symptoms as well, but lack of nutrient absorption may also cause delays in growth and the onset of puberty, vomiting, problems with the enamel on their teeth, and changes in behavior.

Who Can Get Celiac Disease?

Dr. Fasano's 2003 study revealing that 1 in 133 people in the United States suffered from celiac disease was the first time an accurate estimate of celiac disease's prevalence was reported. Since then, awareness of the condition and its symptoms has led some to speculate that it is even more common than that. As Dr. Fasano has noted, celiac disease has a genetic component, in that certain people are predisposed, hereditarily, to get the disease.

FACT

As a genetically transferred disorder, prevalence of celiac disease can skyrocket amongst close relatives. Where the general population has a prevalence of approximately 1 in 133, first-degree relatives of diagnosed individuals have a 1 in 22 chance of also having the disorder. Second-degree relatives have a 1 in 39 chance of having celiac disease.

Genetic predispositions don't automatically mean someone has the condition; in fact, celiac disease can remain largely dormant for many years. But amongst those with a specific genetic makeup, it can appear at any time. Stresses and other environmental factors, including pregnancy, surgery, or even infections, can trigger the onset of severe symptoms. There is no "typical" patient with celiac disease—like many health problems, it does not discriminate, and the prevalence crosses all continents, as well as racial, cultural, and age lines.

Diagnosing Celiac Disease: Blood Tests

Diagnosing celiac disease goes all the way back to Aretaeus of Cappadocia, who used his observations of patients' symptoms to determine their ailment. With time, diagnosis became a matter of observing symptoms and removing wheat from a patient's diet to see if those symptoms went away. These methods have always been vague and subject to misinterpretation, but a diagnostic puzzle could be built by compiling a collage of the patient's clinical and anecdotal symptoms.

In our world of high-tech medical diagnostics, more recent advancements in the scientific understanding of celiac disease have led to better, more complete test methods. Before referring a patient to a gastroenterologist, primary care physicians can perform blood tests. Blood is drawn from a patient on a normal diet and tested for certain immunoglobulin or antibodies that, if present, suggest intolerance to gluten. There is no standardized set of blood tests. Several different tests have been developed and may be administered during the diagnosis process. These are considered screening tests only. While they may foreshadow a diagnosis of celiac disease, they remain inconclusive when used alone.

Anti-Gliadin Antibodies (AGA) Test

Gliadin is one of the component amino acids that, along with *glutenin*, produces gluten. Anti-*gliadin* antibodies are produced when the immune system tries to fight against the *gliadin* as gluten is introduced into the body. This test determines if any IgA class anti-*gliadin* antibodies have been released. This test is reliable; however, other, more reliable tests have been developed and the AGA test is being used less frequently. The other shortfall of this test is that not everyone produces IgA class antibodies under normal circumstances.

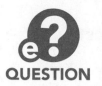

QUESTION

What are immunoglobulins?
Immunoglobulins, part of the molecular machinery that operates within your immune system, are glycoprotein molecules produced by plasma cells. They function as antibodies, binding specifically to one or more invading "antigen" so the immune system can properly deal with it. Immunoglobulins come in five classes: IgA, IgD, IgE, IgG, and IgM. The IgA immunoglobulin is the primary class tested for when celiac disease is suspected. An IgA deficiency affects 3–5 percent of people with celiac disease. In these cases of deficiency, the IgG class immunoglobulin can be used in blood testing.

Endomysial Antibody (EMA) Test

The Endomysial Antibody test checks the blood for the IgA class of endomysial antibodies. Your body develops these antibodies in reaction to ongoing damage to the endomysium, a thin connective tissue layer that covers individual muscle fibers. This test is sensitive and specific; the endomysial antibody is considered the gold standard of antibodies. The EMA test requires examining the blood through microscopy, which leaves the results open to subjectivity and variability between laboratories. Its other main drawback is that it may return false negatives in children under three years of age. Interestingly, in this test, the substance actually being detected is *tissue transglutaminase*, an enzyme released by inflamed intestinal cells in an effort to repair the damage. Despite being released by the intestines in an effort to help, the bizarre immunological response of the celiac's guts is to produce anti-tissue transglutaminase antibodies, which can also be detected in the blood.

QUESTION

What is a "false negative" or "false positive" test result?
A "false negative" test result is one that comes back negative when a disease is actually present. A "false positive" is the opposite—the test is positive, but the disease is not actually present. These can occur for various reasons with many different medical tests.

Anti-tissue Transglutaminase Antibody (anti-tTG) Test

The Anti-tissue Transglutaminase Antibody (anti-tTG) test is considered the most sensitive and specific test for celiac disease. This test also detects the IgA class of anti-tTG antibody. It is inexpensive and rapid, and since it can be performed using laboratory equipment, eliminates the subjectivity introduced when using the EMA test. The anti-tTG test can be performed on a single drop of blood. It can, however, be falsely positive for patients who have another autoimmune condition. It may also return falsely negative results for children under the age of three.

Deamidated Gliadin Peptide (DGP) Antibody Test

The Deamidated Gliadin Peptide (DGP) Antibody test is relatively new and is quickly replacing the Anti-Gliadin Antibody (AGA) test. This test checks a patient's blood for antibodies produced as a result of chemical changes to *gliadin* molecules that have been caused by transglutaminase, the enzyme released by inflamed intestinal cells in an effort to repair the damage. The DGP test is more sensitive and specific and works well for pediatric patients. The Mayo Clinic, in conducting blood testing for celiac disease, uses the Endomysial Antibody (EMA) and Deamidated Gliadin Peptide Antibody tests as secondary or follow-up tests to the primary Anti-tissue Transglutaminase Antibody (anti-tTG) test.

Future Blood Tests

Testing blood serum for antibodies produced when gluten is ingested has long been the primary method used in screening patients for celiac disease. As new research emerges, better tests with greater sensitivity and specificity are being developed. However, these tests remain inconclusive, subject to errors, false negatives, and in some cases, false positives.

Diagnosing Celiac Disease: Biopsies

In diagnosing celiac disease, doctors may use one or all of these blood tests. The results of these tests remain only indicators, though. The only conclusive means to diagnose celiac disease, and the next step for someone who has had the blood testing, is to undergo an intestinal biopsy.

The Intestinal Biopsy

In the effort for a gut with celiac to fight against a gluten attack, a cascade of molecular processes end up harming the affected person's intestines. Remember the villi, the part of the intestinal cells that are akin to fingers projecting into the small intestine? Their normal function is to capture and shunt nutrients across the intestinal wall. In those with celiac disease, however, those villi are damaged as the immune system rampages, and as long as gluten remains present in the diet, they won't grow back.

Observing this damage to the villi is the only way to conclusively arrive at a diagnosis of celiac disease. Villi are microscopic structures and the only way to properly observe them is by bringing a sample outside the body. That's where the intestinal biopsy comes in. A biopsy is the removal and diagnostic study of tissue from a living body. Biopsies are routinely conducted for a variety of medical reasons, on a variety of the body's organs. Intestinal biopsies, also known as endoscopic biopsies, are conducted by obtaining tissue from the upper part of the small intestine.

How It Works

An endoscope, a long tube with a camera on the end, is first inserted through the patient's mouth. The doctor carefully feeds the tube through the esophagus and into the stomach. Once in the stomach, the doctor uses the image from the endoscope, displayed on a monitor, to assess any other problems that may exist. He then finds the entryway to the small intestine. This area is referred to as the duodenum and may appear normal during the endoscopic exam.

To remove the tissue needed for examination, the doctor inserts a small surgical instrument through the endoscope tube and takes samples from several areas. The surgical instrument grasps a small portion of the intestine and, in the correct orientation, slices a piece away. The tissue samples must be sliced in the correct orientation so that the pathologist viewing the samples under a microscope can make a proper diagnosis. The cuts are not deep, and they are intended only to remove a small cellular sample, not puncture the intestine. There are no nerve endings in the intestine, making the biopsy a virtually pain-free procedure.

ALERT

Despite all the methods available for diagnosing celiac disease, the fact that the symptoms so closely match other conditions makes the screening process difficult and often a long, protracted process that can span several years. Studies by celiac associations have shown that many people had to seek out the help of three or more doctors, over the course of several years, before finally being diagnosed.

The surgical procedure can be performed while under general anaesthetic, and—not counting preparation and recovery from anaesthetic—is a relatively quick procedure, lasting less than twenty minutes. If you have been scheduled for a biopsy, do not go on a gluten-free diet, as the villi may begin to heal and the biopsy test could return a false negative result.

Treating Celiac Disease

The diagnosis of celiac disease might be modern and high-tech, but its treatment is almost ancient and can be summed up in one simple word: diet. The only known way to treat celiac disease is with a strict adherence to a gluten-free diet. Only by removing the environmental trigger—gluten—will the harmful immunologic responses in the gut stop. Only by removing gluten will the intestines be allowed to begin the process of healing themselves. It's a fact that, at this point, there is no other way. But that doesn't mean there will never be another form of treatment.

The Latest Research

Dr. Alessio Fasano, whose team identified that gluten, genetic susceptibility, and a leaky gut were the three factors that combine to produce celiac disease, has also suggested that there may be other ways to treat the disease. Dr. Fasano has proposed that, since eliminating one leg in the triangle—gluten—solves the problem, maybe disrupting one of the other elements in the process may also offer a treatment option.

Several therapies are currently under development:

1. One is exploring an orally administered protein-enzyme designed to break down gluten completely so it is no longer resistant to digestion.
2. Other pharmaceutical companies are investigating ways to inhibit tissue transglutaminase to prevent the biochemical modifications they produce in gluten in the gut.
3. An Australian company is working on developing a vaccine that would be administered to a patient in an effort to force the immune system to tolerate gluten.

4. Dr. Fasano himself cofounded a company that is researching medications to prevent the junctions between intestinal cells from opening. He is no longer directly involved in that company's work, but maintains an arms-length relationship as a scientific adviser. Their product has actually been tested in two human trials in an effort to determine tolerability, side effects, and treatment effectiveness. These tests have shown some very promising results.

As head of the University of Maryland's Center for Celiac Research, Dr. Fasano is leading teams of researchers who are working to improve the lives of celiac patients and others negatively affected by gluten. His team has already identified the different mechanisms leading to gluten sensitivity and celiac disease, and how the two are part of a spectrum of gluten-related disorders. They are currently working on a study to determine if delaying the introduction of gluten into the diets of genetically susceptible babies will help prevent the onset of celiac disease in these infants. They already have more than 750 babies, worldwide, enrolled in this study.

Women and Celiac Disease

Women with celiac disease are more likely to report symptoms of depression and disordered eating, despite being on a gluten-free diet. This is from researchers at Penn State, Syracuse University, and Drexel University in the United States. The study was conducted online and gauged the emotional experiences of 177 American women over the age of eighteen who have been diagnosed with celiac disease. Although the study found that most participants adhered to a gluten-free diet and managed their illness well, they still reported higher rates of stress, depression, and dissatisfaction with their body image than the general population. The researchers hope that, in the future, treatments will involve the physical symptoms while also addressing these accompanying psychological, social, and behavioral aspects.

A Columbia University study by the Center for Women's Reproductive Care indicated that women with unexplained infertility were more likely to suffer from undiagnosed celiac disease. This small study is far from conclusive, but the four subjects who, through the process of the study, were diagnosed and embarked on a gluten-free diet, all became pregnant within a year of diagnosis.

Is There a Cure Coming?

Other efforts to find new treatments, or possibly even a cure, are ongoing. The University of Chicago's Celiac Disease Center website boldly proclaims, "We seek to cure celiac disease by 2026." How do they plan on accomplishing that? "Intensive, focused research." The University of Chicago's goal is being led by Bana Jabri, MD, PhD. Her team is working with human and mouse-model subjects to better understand how celiac disease works on the molecular level. Recently, Dr. Jabri published research that added to that understanding. Her team was able to identify two chemical signals, interleukin 15 (IL-15) and retinoic acid—a derivative of vitamin A that triggers the inflammatory response to gluten. By blocking IL-15 in their mouse model, the team was able to prevent the development of the disease.

FACT

Finding cures for diseases requires a model to study—a lab rat, if you will. In reality, lab *mice* are most often used. No mouse model currently exists that completely replicates celiac disease, so Dr. Jabri's team is earnestly working on the first. They are breeding multiple strains of genetically modified mice, each exhibiting one of the characteristics of celiac disease, and then will breed the strains together in hopes of producing a strain that exhibits all the necessary characteristics.

The University of Chicago's goal of curing celiac disease by 2026 is noble and should give people living with celiac disease some hope. This ancient disease with a simple treatment is being investigated with very modern, very high-tech procedures by some of the brightest scientific minds of our day. These efforts need to be supported and monitored so that one day research into celiac disease will no longer be necessary.

CHAPTER 3

Gluten-Free for Other Reasons

Gluten is an environmental trigger that, in susceptible individuals, causes the chain reaction of autoimmunity in the gut that leads to celiac disease. But as doctors and scientists learn more about how gluten affects the body, they are finding a wide spectrum of disorders that are induced or influenced by gluten. Maintaining a gluten-free diet may help alleviate some of the symptoms in these disorders. Some people may choose to go gluten-free for still other reasons as well, but there are also times when it might not be the best choice.

The Spectrum

In 2011, a panel of fifteen experts convened in London to establish a medical consensus on the proper wording for gluten-related disorders. The group, led by Dr. Alessio Fasano, included colleagues from research centers in the United States, Italy, Argentina, Slovenia, Finland, the UK, and Germany. Dr. Schär, the leading producer of gluten-free food, sponsored the work by this global body of experts. Each panelist was assigned a specific topic with a goal to developing definitions, classifications, and diagnostic algorithms for the variety of gluten-induced disorders. The panelist's work represents a clear starting point for understanding the differences and similarities between autoimmune reactions, allergic reactions, and immune-mediated reactions to gluten. Following are some summaries of what they found.

Celiac Disease

Celiac disease is an autoimmune reaction to gluten characterized by a genetic susceptibility in affected individuals. Recent studies indicate the disease is trending upward in prevalence. This trend is expected to continue and might be attributed to the increasing worldwide consumption of wheat. What was once a disease that mainly affected people of European descent has begun to affect populations in Africa and Asia as their diets become more Westernized.

Dermatitis Herpetiformis

Dermatitis Herpetiformis (DH) is the manifestation of celiac disease on the skin of affected individuals. Blistering rashes form and may or may not be accompanied by intestinal symptoms. Incidence of gastrointestinal problems in patients with DH is approximately 10 percent, yet many do show damage to the intestinal villi. Doctors are not sure why this happens. Like celiac disease, DH is most prevalent or common amongst descendants of European origin. The rates of DH are much lower than celiac disease, with current estimates at one in 10,000. The manifestation of DH, like celiac disease, can occur at any age but is most common around the time of adulthood to midlife and is more common in men than in women.

No one knows what links the intestinal and skin lesions in Dermatitis Herpetiformis, but antibodies are present in the skin and the rash itself is gluten-sensitive. Patients develop skin abnormalities that change and develop and may rupture. Once dry, these areas scab over and produce itching and burning on the surface of the skin. In over 90 percent of cases, the rash that develops follows a characteristic distribution along the elbows and upper forearms. Rashes may also develop on the buttocks, knees, shoulders, face, neck, and scalp. In a small quantity of cases, the rash is intermittent; in most, however, it is a constant problem.

To diagnose DH, pathologists test for the same blood antibodies as in celiac disease and by checking for IgA antibodies in areas of the skin where the rash hasn't formed or expressed itself. Biopsies from those areas are examined for a particular granular or fibular deposit of IgA antibodies. Diagnosing DH removes the need for an intestinal biopsy, as the skin condition is considered indirect evidence of bowel damage.

Treatment for DH is the same as for celiac disease, despite the fact that sufferers may not have any digestive problems or their intestines appear normal.

Gluten Ataxia

Ataxia is the loss of coordination of the muscles, especially in the extremities. It is another autoimmune response to gluten. Ataxia can occur sporadically for other reasons, but studies have shown that the introduction of gluten into the intestine can account for a high percentage—approximately 23 percent—of cases.

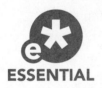

ESSENTIAL

One recent study showed that injecting mice with anti-tissue Transglutaminase (anti-tTG) derived from patient blood serum can cause ataxia in the subject mice. This study appears to provide evidence that anti-tTG antibodies compromise certain neuronal functions in the brain. This would seem to indicate that the onset of ataxia is independent of the immune system's response to gluten, but is directly dependent on the chemical products of the immune response, i.e., anti-tTG antibodies.

In gluten ataxia, chemical reactions and interactions among antibodies, gluten proteins, and certain cells are believed to be the cause. Doctors have found deposits of transglutaminase antibodies around brain vessels in the cerebellum, pons, and medulla regions of the brain, indicating a connection between ataxia and gluten consumption.

The average age at the onset of gluten ataxia is fifty-three years, suggesting it is more of a problem at mid–late life. Gluten ataxia can affect eyes, mobility, and limb movement, but often there is little or no evidence of intestinal damage after undergoing a biopsy. Gluten ataxia can even lead to brain damage, with magnetic resonance imaging showing cerebellar atrophy.

Diagnosing gluten ataxia is a bit trickier than diagnosing celiac disease or Dermatitis Herpetiformis. The current recommendation is to perform a more comprehensive antibody test of sample blood. Patients need to be tested for both IgG and IgA class antibodies, as well as several different types of antibodies. If these tests are positive, then an intestinal biopsy should be performed merely to determine if any damage has occurred. If a patient is positive for these antibodies and no other reason for the ataxia exists, they must begin a gluten-free diet with physician follow-up to ensure the ataxia has stabilized or improved. It may take up to a year before a doctor determines that a patient does indeed suffer from gluten ataxia.

Wheat Allergy

Allergic reactions to wheat also involve immunologic reactions to wheat proteins. However, in wheat allergies, symptoms begin in a matter of minutes to hours after exposure to gluten. Allergic reactions can occur on the skin, in the gastrointestinal tract, or in the respiratory tract and will be largely dependent on the route by which the allergen enters or contacts the body. Occupational asthma, also known as baker's asthma, is perhaps the most common allergic reaction to wheat. Caused by the inhalation of wheat dust or the dust of other cereal flours, baker's asthma is one of the most prevalent occupational allergies. Fortunately, baker's asthma mostly affects those in the baking industry. A Polish study showed that respiratory symptoms increase in the number of affected apprentices the longer they are exposed to wheat dust.

Baker's asthma is not readily treated by a gluten-free diet; however, staying away from gluten and adopting a gluten-free lifestyle may be required to ensure allergic reactions are not triggered.

If developed as a food allergy, along the lines of more traditional food allergies, like peanuts or seafood, ingested wheat can cause anaphylaxis, dermatitis, and hives.

Doctors diagnose wheat allergies through the use of skin-prick tests and by testing for IgE class antibodies. These are not conclusive tests, with predictive values less than 75 percent, due to complications from grass pollen; however, they offer a starting point. Final diagnosis often requires what is known as an "oral food challenge." None of the studies conducted thus far have shown that the blood serum IgG antibody tests used in diagnosing celiac disease can be used to diagnose wheat allergy.

Nonceliac Gluten Sensitivity

Celiac disease is the specific autoimmune response to the introduction of gluten into the small intestine. Since the autoimmunity causes damage to the intestine, the clinical name for what is commonly known as celiac disease is *gluten-induced enteropathy*. As celiac disease is studied more, anecdotal and scientific evidence that gluten can induce a whole spectrum of medical health issues, without the patient experiencing celiac disease, is growing. This spectrum includes nonceliac gluten sensitivity.

Although gluten sensitivity is not considered a disease, it can trigger other diseases, including rheumatoid arthritis, fibromyalgia, osteoporosis, and a variety of neurological disorders. Here are a few conditions that may be associated with a gluten sensitivity:

- Headaches
- Anxiety
- Attention deficit
- Ataxia
- Epilepsy
- Sleep disorders
- Developmental delays
- Encephalopathy
- Hypoperfusion
- Hypotonia

Gluten sensitivity is not the sole cause of these conditions and it is also not easily diagnosed. There are no "biomarkers" that can be observed in a laboratory setting to definitively conclude a sensitivity to gluten. Therefore, diagnosis is restricted to removing gluten from the diet, followed by a physician evaluation to determine if health has improved.

How Gluten-Free Living Can Help Other Problems

Living gluten-free is necessary for some—such as people with diagnosed celiac disease or gluten sensitivity—but there are a variety of health issues that may also be helped by removing wheat and other cereal crops from the diet. The range of issues helped by eliminating gluten is diverse and, at times, surprising. Everything from psychological problems to mobility issues to other autoimmune disorders may benefit from, if not be effectively managed by, a gluten-free diet.

Autism

The term "autism" is used to identify a specific condition or syndrome, as well as a broad range of related disorders. Medical professionals generally agree that a full-blown case of autism spectrum disorder involves three related disorders or impairments. People with autism have:

- Difficulty with social interaction
- Problems with communication and language usage
- Limited development of play and imagination, characterized by repetitive behavior patterns

Some people have only one of the symptoms while others may have any combination of two.

No one knows exactly what causes autism, but it is essentially a disorder of the development of brain functions in which a variety of factors are believed to be involved. Autism is associated with other neurological disorders, brain abnormalities, and chemical imbalances, and there is some evidence that it may also be a genetic condition. One theory, the opioid-excess hypothesis, suggests that autism is caused, in part, by the incomplete breakdown and absorption of protein peptides with opioid activity.

QUESTION

What are peptides and opioids?
A peptide is a protein compound containing two or more amino acids in which one group, known as the carboxyl, is attached to another group, known as the amino group. Opioids are any naturally occurring substance that causes effects similar to opium.

In the case of autism, the offending protein peptides come from two main sources, gluten and casein, a protein derived from dairy products. Studies have shown that many children with autism who also experienced gastrointestinal symptoms when exposed to gluten and casein benefited from a diet change—when they were placed on a gluten- and casein-free diet, they showed dramatic improvements in behaviors associated with the spectrum of autism, physiological symptoms, and social behaviors.

It's important to note that the greatest benefits come when gluten and casein are completely eliminated from the diet over a long term. Only reducing or removing one source (gluten or casein), or failure to follow through for the long term, produced less beneficial results.

Schizophrenia

Schizophrenia is a mental illness, usually developing in late adolescence or early adulthood. It is characterized by five major symptoms:

- Delusions
- Hallucinations
- Bizarre behavior
- Disorganized speech
- A variety of negative symptoms, including diminished cognitive functioning

The root words *schizo* and *phrene* are Greek for "split" and "mind" and clearly describe the fragmented thinking associated with this disorder. The cause of schizophrenia is also a mystery since no one is sure what causes it, and it can only be classified by observing the symptoms.

Treatments for schizophrenia often follow the traditional pattern for mental disease and disorders. These include medication, therapy, and hospitalization. Doctors also try to educate the patient and their family about managing the disorder and in some cases patients are helped by attending support groups or day-treatment programs. One interesting development that is beginning to emerge is how a gluten-free diet can benefit people with schizophrenia.

FACT

It appears that children of mothers with gluten sensitivity have a higher risk of developing mental disorders including schizophrenia. The study, by the Karolinska Institutet in Sweden and Johns Hopkins University, was the first to identify maternal food sensitivity as the prime suspect in the development of these disorders later in life.

Results of adopting a gluten-free diet have been mixed among published studies dealing with schizophrenia. In one study by Johns Hopkins Bloomberg School of Public Health, a review of the available literature showed that some patients experienced "a drastic reduction, if not full remission, of schizophrenic symptoms" after they embarked on a gluten-free diet. These positive results only occurred in a subset of patients, meaning not everyone with schizophrenia would necessarily benefit from a gluten-free diet. The conclusion also stated that more studies are required to try and establish what mechanisms link gluten and schizophrenia.

Rheumatoid Arthritis

Rheumatoid arthritis is the chronic inflammation of the joints. It is an autoimmune reaction—something it has in common with celiac disease. However, in rheumatoid arthritis, the body's immune system attacks the thin membrane, known as the synovium, which lines the joints. Rheumatoid arthritis causes pain and inflammation and may result in joint damage. Joints most affected include hands, wrists, elbows, feet, ankles, and knees.

The cause of rheumatoid arthritis is also unknown, but links to genetics and environmental factors—two more things in common with celiac disease—have long been suspected. Diagnosing rheumatoid arthritis is based largely on physical examination and medical history.

There are not many scientific studies that have been conducted to look into the link between gluten and rheumatoid arthritis. Fewer studies have been conducted on the effects of a gluten-free diet, but ample anecdotal evidence exists to suggest that a gluten-free diet may help dramatically reduce pain and other symptoms in some patients. One study conducted by researchers based in Guadalajara, Mexico, and published in 2010, concluded that people initially diagnosed with rheumatoid arthritis may, in fact, be misdiagnosed celiac patients.

Osteoporosis

Osteoporosis is a disease that causes low bone mass and the loss or deterioration of bone density. The deterioration happens silently, without symptoms, and can result in fragile bones that are easily broken. Rates of fracture due to osteoporosis vary between genders. Estimates place men at a 1 in 5 chance for fracture and women at 1 in 3 during their lifetimes.

ALERT

Fractures due to osteoporosis are so common among all groups with the condition that their occurrence outnumbers the incidence of heart attack, stroke, and breast cancer combined. Considered a pediatric disease with geriatric consequences, meaning the problem starts in childhood but only impacts the sufferer later in life, statistics show that about 80 percent of fractures in people over the age of sixty are related to osteoporosis.

Like the other diseases examined thus far, osteoporosis has no single cause, at least not one that has been identified. Gluten sensitivity and celiac disease are considered high risk factors for developing osteoporosis. Several studies have suggested a link between malabsorption of minerals due to celiac disease and osteoporosis. But there is another possible connection as well. In some cases, nonceliac gluten intolerance, which can't be tested for in the way celiac disease can, has been ruled the culprit in bone density loss. In these cases, a diet free of gluten reversed the effects of bone tissue loss.

Type 1 Diabetes

Physical energy for your body comes from when the food you eat is converted into glucose. That glucose is transported and regulated through the blood by the hormone insulin. In type 1 diabetes, the insulin-producing organ, the pancreas, fails to produce insulin. Without the insulin regulation, glucose builds up and does not get converted to energy.

Like many other diseases, the cause of type 1 diabetes remains unknown. It is not preventable and, like celiac disease and so many other conditions, is an autoimmune disease. In a manner similar to celiac disease, the body's immune system produces antibodies that attack the pancreas. Also like celiac disease, genetic and environmental factors play a role in triggering the onset. While medical professionals admit that environmental factors like pathogens, toxins, drugs, and perhaps most important, food components contribute to the development of the disease, the generally accepted prime suspect is viral infections. At least one study from 2009 has concluded a possible link between wheat "polypeptides" (chains of amino acids) and the immune system response that leads to type 1 diabetes.

ESSENTIAL

Identical twins have the same genetic susceptibility to type 1 diabetes. But studies have shown that rates of disease incidence between twins are not equal. To put it another way, one identical twin may get type 1 diabetes and one may not. The difference isn't genetics, so it must be environment.

Despite not knowing the exact cause of diabetes, it can be clinically diagnosed using any one, or combination, of three methods. The first method involves fasting for eight hours and drawing blood to measure the amount of glucose present. The second method is similar; the patient fasts for eight hours and then drinks a glucose-based beverage. After two hours, blood is drawn and the amount of glucose present is measured. The third method draws blood regardless of when the person last ate and checks the level of glucose. The first two tests also work to diagnose prediabetes.

Therapy for this disease may include insulin or other prescribed medications, adopting a healthy diet, and increased physical activity. There is no controversy over the fact that people with type 1 diabetes have an increased risk for celiac disease. Evidence is beginning to mount that suggests that diabetes may in fact be a result of gluten sensitivity. A 2009 study by researchers at the Ottawa Hospital Research Institute in Canada examined the immune response to wheat peptides in patients with type 1 diabetes. Their results raised the possibility that wheat could, in fact, be the primary dietary trigger in the development of type 1 diabetes. Treating diabetes already requires adopting a healthy diet, which may be a great time to eliminate gluten from the diet as well.

Gluten-Free for Weight Loss?

While exercise plays an important role in a weight-loss journey, adopting a healthy diet is also necessary to attain one's desired weight. Going gluten-free is certainly a change in diet, but whether it works as a "weight loss diet" is questionable. But since more celebrities are promoting a gluten-free lifestyle, it's important to examine the issue of weight loss while going gluten-free very carefully.

Many people with celiac disease have experienced weight loss after going gluten-free, but many have also experienced weight gain. There is considerable debate on both sides of the issue, but one thing is clear: It's as easy to consume empty calories while eating gluten-free as it is on an unrestricted diet.

Going gluten-free will certainly eliminate the amount of wheat-based carbohydrates in your diet, but chances are, those carbohydrates will be replaced with noncereal carbohydrates. Take pasta, for example. There are gluten-free rice and corn-based pastas available, so a nice dish of spaghetti and meat sauce, made with corn pasta and a good, thick gluten-free sauce, will still contain a high amount of dietary carbohydrates. Since most gluten-free pasta contains very low fiber compared to whole-wheat pasta, the net nutritional value of the gluten-free meal may actually be worse. This scenario can be repeated with many other gluten-free replacement foods and must be kept in mind when making meal-planning choices.

Weight loss while on a gluten-free diet is often associated more with food restrictions than with any unique weight loss properties associated with a gluten-free diet. People avoiding gluten have limited choices when dining out, forcing them away from deep-fried foods and toward the salad menu. Many gluten-free snack foods are made with "all-natural" ingredients, but if the ingredients contain high volumes of calories or fat, it doesn't really matter if they are natural if weight loss is the goal. The gluten-free diet is unique in that it is started, usually, for chronic medical reasons.

Gluten-Free for Anti-Inflammation

While the weight-loss potential of a gluten-free diet is questionable, its effects on inflammation are almost overwhelming. Doctors already know that gluten-induced reactions can cause inflammation in the intestine, and that there is a strong link between gluten and rheumatoid arthritis, the inflammation of the synovium. There is also ample evidence that gluten can trigger a whole host of other inflammatory conditions in the body.

Lupus is an autoimmune disorder that turns the body's immune system against many of its different tissues. Some of the most common symptoms include painful or swollen joints, unexplained fever, skin rashes, and kidney problems. The condition is generally treated with medications, but one preliminary study from 2004 suggests that a gluten-free diet may be the answer.

FACT

The full clinical name for lupus is *systemic lupus erythematosus* (SLE). It is a chronic condition that, if untreated, can prove fatal. The name of the disease is derived from the Latin word "lupus," which means "wolf," and "erythematosus," which means redness. This Latin word-picture is derived from the reddish lesions, similar in appearance to a wolf bite, which appear on the faces of people with severe symptoms.

There are a variety of other inflammatory conditions that have been linked to gluten intake. Bursitis, irritable bowel syndrome, Crohn's disease, and ulcerative colitis are all autoimmune and inflammatory conditions that, some sufferers say, can be triggered by the ingestion of gluten. Most of the inflammation due to gluten ingestion goes back to how the intestines respond to the introduction of gluten. The cyclone of immune responses that swirls like a hurricane through the gut of a susceptible individual causes the tight junctions between the cells of the intestinal lining to open up producing a "leaky gut." Without these tight junctions, gluten strands and other invasive molecules can penetrate the barrier into the tissues below. This further activates the immune system, one consequence of which is the production of oxidants, which cause irritation and inflammation in places far away from the gut that originally triggered them.

Feeling Better Overall

It's not hard to see that when you consider celiac disease, wheat allergies, the entire spectrum of gluten sensitivity, and many autoimmune and inflammatory disorders, there are many reasons to go gluten-free. Knowing that all these conditions might be related to gluten, and knowing that gluten is a very real environmental trigger that is extremely common in the standard American diet, going gluten-free might just be the answer to feeling better overall.

Anytime a doctor says the words "autoimmune disorder," and there is no known cause for the condition, consider gluten as the source and ask about the possibility of treating it with a gluten-free diet. Likewise, if you are experiencing ongoing unexplained gastrointestinal symptoms, ask your doctor if a gluten-free diet might help you. There is nothing wrong with making inquiries that your doctor may have never considered before, if it will mean feeling better overall.

Gluten-Free Kids

Many autoimmune conditions present themselves in young patients while they are still considered pediatric. For example, a form of rheumatoid arthritis, called juvenile idiopathic arthritis (JIA), can appear in children as young as six months old up to around age 16. Other than the suspicion of bacteria and viruses, JIA, like type 1 diabetes, is an autoimmune condition that has no known cause. Although no direct link to gluten has been established, scientists know that the incidence of celiac disease is higher in children with autoimmune disorders like JIA and Type 1 diabetes. This leads some doctors to conclude that it may be a consequence of untreated celiac disease. Even children without these serious conditions can benefit from a gluten-free diet, especially if they suffer from attention deficit hyperactivity disorder or autism.

You might want to ask your child's doctor about a gluten-free diet if he or she is suffering from behavioral or digestive problems for which doctors are unable to find an explanation. If eliminating gluten from a child's diet helps improve their condition, continue to keep in touch with the child's doctor to see if that development helps open up other diagnoses possibilities and to discuss the viability of going gluten-free as a long-term solution. If you are comfortable doing so, share your experience with the wider gluten-free community as well. Every piece of evidence, whether scientific or anecdotal, has the potential to help others who may be experiencing similar problems with their children.

The Wrong Reasons to Go Gluten-Free

There are many reasons to adopt a gluten-free diet. Certainly a diagnosis of celiac disease is not only a good reason, but a firm prescription. The entire spectrum of nonceliac gluten sensitivity, whether diagnosed or suspected, provides another very strong reason. But are there wrong reasons to go gluten-free?

If you suspect that you have celiac disease, going gluten-free prior to a proper diagnosis with intestinal biopsy is definitely a bad idea. Eliminating gluten from your diet before undergoing the procedure may allow your gut enough time to heal so the pathologist won't be able to make a correct diagnosis.

With dubious claims and little supporting scientific evidence, going gluten-free for weight loss purposes is also a bad idea. Don't get trapped in any kind of fad or swept into a lifestyle because of something a celebrity is doing. Instead, spend the time investigating, and consulting with your health care providers, to make sure the gluten-free lifestyle is the right choice for you.

Care should be taken when making any major lifestyle change. The spectrum of gluten-induced sensitivity is ever-widening, providing more reasons to go gluten-free all the time. But there may also be wrong reasons to go gluten-free, depending on your personal health situation, and that's where careful exploration of the subject is essential to making the right choice and the proper decision for your health and the health of your family. In all cases, the decision to eat gluten-free should not be made without consultation with a healthcare professional.

CHAPTER 4

Starting a Gluten-Free Diet

Starting a gluten-free diet is not something to take lightly. There are many reasons to consider a gluten-free diet, with the primary one being a recommendation by a physician. Once you've made the choice, the real work begins. Not only do you need to design an entirely new meal plan and adapt your favorite recipes so you can continue to enjoy them, you need to deal with explaining your diet to others. While adopting a gluten-free lifestyle, you also need to manage the physical and psychological effects of withdrawing gluten from your diet and any complications that adhering to a stricter diet, like vegetarian or vegan, can cause.

Is a Gluten-Free Diet Right for You?

Is a gluten-free diet right for you? It depends. Certainly, if you are diagnosed with celiac disease through a biopsy, the choice has been made for you. Living gluten-free is no longer an option; it's mandatory to regain and sustain your health. It is the only long-term treatment option, currently available, for treating celiac disease and promoting the healing your body needs in the wake of the ravages gluten has wrought on your intestine.

If a doctor has not prescribed a gluten-free diet, but you suspect that eliminating gluten from your diet will help you, or someone close to you, then the choice is less distinct. The wide spectrum of disorders associated with gluten's toxicity in the human body doesn't require eliminating gluten like celiac disease does, but, in the interests of health and well-being, it might be the right thing to do. So then the questions become, do you eliminate all gluten entirely, or just a small amount? And do you eliminate it all at once, or do you work at reducing the amount of gluten in your diet slowly?

If you choose to eliminate gluten for some other reason, personal choice, in support of someone else, or because of fitness goals, then these same questions may apply, but the pace at which you answer them are open to your own timeline. As mentioned in the previous chapter, consult with your doctor before adopting a nonprescribed gluten-free diet.

Placing the mandatory reason—celiac disease—aside for a moment, consider the choice to go gluten-free for other reasons. Do you have the commitment and resources to adopt a gluten-free lifestyle? This may be easier to answer once fully immersed in the diet and you've noticed improvements in your health, but until then it may take will power, stamina, and a rock solid plan to achieve your goals.

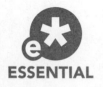

ESSENTIAL

Gluten-free "convenience" foods (e.g., prepared foods and snacks) are becoming more and more common on the shelves of your favorite grocery stores. The relatively small market for these products is growing, but they remain more costly than their gluten-containing equivalents. Taking these additional costs into consideration is very important when deciding if a gluten-free diet is right for you.

While trying to determine if a gluten-free diet is right for you, it might be helpful to make a list of pros and cons to help you in your evaluation. Discussing the idea with others who have already adopted a gluten-free lifestyle, or consulting a dietician, may also prove beneficial in your decision-making process.

Once you've made the decision to embrace a gluten-free lifestyle, or the decision is made for you by your medical condition, you will need to begin the real work. It will take considerable thought, effort, and planning.

A Twenty-Four-Hour Job—at First

In the long term, gluten-free living will not be a twenty-four-hour job. But at the beginning, as you approach each day wondering how you are going to prepare safe meals for breakfast, lunch, and supper, it may feel like one. If you factor in the needs of family or loved ones, or how you will handle business and social situations, the feeling that you are on the clock twenty-four-seven, looking after your health, will increase.

Perhaps the best thing to do is understand this and decide that in the beginning, you must allow your new gluten-free life to occupy as much of your time as necessary. It is your health, after all. Although slower acting and less perceptible than more acute diseases, celiac disease is a serious condition. No one would fault someone with a more serious illness if, after their initial diagnosis, they spend a considerable amount of time occupied with contemplating the treatment options and lifestyle changes that will be necessary for their complete recovery.

Once you've spent the time figuring out your plan, tested the waters on some products or recipes, and discussed your diet with those around you, the pressure will ease. Even though this is when the day-to-day work of living gluten-free will actually begin, the initial overwhelming feeling of the twenty-four-hour job will begin to subside. Developing any new routine will require dedication and discipline at first, but eventually it will become, well, routine. Living gluten-free is no different. Eventually, it will become your new "normal."

Try a Few Recipes

In the case of celiac disease, beginning a gluten-free diet is a matter of going cold turkey. There really is no room for a gradual reduction. It's the steepest, most dramatic learning curve associated with beginning a gluten-free life. One day, you ate toast and coffee for breakfast before going to the hospital for your biopsy. The next day, you literally eliminate all gluten from your life. If you've prepared well, you can still have toast and coffee for breakfast on this second day, but it will have to be with gluten-free bread.

ALERT

Remember, if you are being tested for celiac disease, you have to continue eating a diet that contains gluten until after the biopsy, even if the blood work comes back positive. Once the biopsy is done, though, and you are waiting on the results from your doctor, you can spend some time considering gluten-free foods.

Start with Naturally Gluten-Free Foods

It might be best, at this early stage, to stick to a few naturally gluten-free recipes. This will not be the time to learn to bake gluten-free bread, which can be tricky at first. Try some dishes that don't rely heavily on bread or flour, or recipes where any flour can be easily substituted. Grilled steak and a baked potato is a great example of a classic meal that doesn't naturally contain any gluten. Pass on the garlic bread, and prepare a nice big garden salad or other vegetable side dish and you've just had one of the best gluten-free meals available. Other options include baking a ham or roasting a chicken and serving it with corn.

Moving On

Many standard comfort foods and dishes can be made naturally gluten-free. If you love Italian food, you can now start to experiment with different gluten-free pasta. Make gluten-free lasagna. Use your favorite recipe, double-checking that all purchased sauces and spices are indeed gluten-free, and replace the normal lasagna noodles with gluten-free lasagna noodles. Be sure to follow the instructions on the box for cooking the noodles.

FACT

Most gluten-free pasta is made with either rice flour or corn flour. Gluten-free pasta has different cooking times from regular wheat-based pasta and may need to be handled more delicately when being rinsed in a colander. Be sure to read and follow the instructions on the pasta package.

You can also try gluten-free spaghetti and fettuccini noodles with your favorite meat, marinara, or Alfredo sauce. Gluten-free pasta does taste differently from wheat-based pasta, but the rich, thick aromas, and wonderful textures of Italian sauces, make the difference undetectable to most people.

Other ethnic foods to try include Mexican and Chinese. Chicken tacos using corn tortillas, served with refried beans, corn chips, salsa, and guacamole, makes a great gluten-free meal. So does stir-fried vegetables served over rice vermicelli for the Chinese food lover. Just double-check your ingredients ahead of time to make sure they are gluten-free.

More Advanced Options

As you get comfortable with traditional recipes that are easy to convert by eliminating or switching an ingredient or two, you can begin to expand into more difficult territory. If you were a baker before, there's no reason to stop now. Gluten-free baking can produce great quality cookies, cakes, and breads that are almost indistinguishable from standard baked goods. It is best to ease into gluten-free baking, by trying a few recipes at first, as you will need to stock up on new ingredients and figure out which flours you prefer to use.

If you have a diagnosed child with a birthday coming up, birthday cake or cupcakes should be high on the list of recipes to try. Cakes are a great place to start. If they don't turn out perfectly smooth or even on top, use a generous amount of frosting and sprinkles to disguise the imperfections.

Emotional Effects of Removing Gluten from Your Diet

What happens when gluten is removed from the diet varies from person to person. For some, the thought immediately produces anxiety. Wheat and other cereal crops are so abundant and convenient, and used so often in modern food preparation, that even thinking about avoiding them can cause people to begin worrying. For others, it may produce defiance. Love for certain foods and a desire to resist changing their lifestyle may put them in direct conflict with the need to begin a gluten-free lifestyle.

Removing gluten may also produce a new preoccupation with food. Preparation and planning to make sure you have access to safe, nutritious food in all situations may prompt some people to begin thinking about food in a context that they never have before. You may even dream about food or whether or not something contains gluten. Many people have startled themselves awake after dreaming they accidentally ingested gluten. Preoccupation with the food you are consuming, and whether it contains gluten or not, will always be present in your conscious thoughts and your subconscious.

One other major factor to consider is the effect on your grocery budget. Processed gluten-free food and individual ingredients are still niche market items, making them more expensive than comparable food items.

The important thing to remember is that despite the psychological and financial effects, removing gluten is still the right thing to do. Apprehension and lifestyle adjustments aside, eliminating gluten is necessary for your body to begin healing, and many of these negative, initial consequences will quickly be overshadowed by the improvements in overall health and well-being.

Physical Side Effects and Gluten Detox

For people with celiac disease, or those suffering from the broad spectrum of gluten-induced sensitivities, gluten is a toxic protein. Ingesting it can produce either immediate or delayed reactions or health problems. Eliminating gluten from the diet, in these cases, is a very good idea, and it may be essential for full health recovery. Yet people can still experience physical side effects during the process of detoxifying their body from gluten.

While there are very few, possibly no, scientific studies that have investigated what happens physiologically to a person who is detoxifying their body of gluten, there is much anecdotal evidence that it may produce similar results as detoxifying from other toxins, like drugs and alcohol.

Irritability and changes in mood are two of the most common and dramatic results of the detoxification process. This may be linked to the opioid-binding nature of gluten peptides. Other chemical changes in the body resulting from the elimination of gluten may also account for some of these effects. Pile the chemical shifts in the body on top of cravings for, and denial of, favorite foods, and detoxification can become a volatile mix that can be difficult to handle at times.

Moving to a gluten-free diet is a disrupting change in lifestyle. Many of the symptoms associated with eliminating gluten are psychological and some are physiological. It is important to remember that the whole reason to go gluten-free is to return your body to its normal functions. It may be a new normal that you are returning to, but it will become normal. As you heal and progress through the process, it will also become a very healthy and enjoyable normal. Planning properly and having support in place to help deal with the variety of psychological and physiological problems associated with shifting your lifestyle to gluten-free will help minimize the impact that the symptoms of gluten detoxification will throw at you.

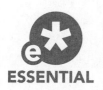

ESSENTIAL

Many support options are available to help you through the transition to a gluten-free lifestyle. Support websites and blogs feature articles on getting started, and contain listings for local face-to-face support groups (see Appendix C for more information). Also, speak to your family doctor and request a referral to a nutritionist to assist you during this transition.

Gluten-Free Vegans and Vegetarians

Vegans and vegetarians are already obeying a strict dietary code. There are many different reasons one might begin a vegetarian diet; health, morality, and religious choice may all play a part in making that decision. Someone who has already put that much thought into the food they regularly eat is well positioned to take the necessary steps to begin a gluten-free lifestyle. But vegetarians will also encounter several problems when shifting to a gluten-free diet.

Wheat comes from a plant, making it completely vegan. It is very versatile in the diet and used in many products. Wheat is also highly nutritious, adding a significant amount of nutrients, including dietary fiber, protein, vitamins, and other minerals to a vegetarian's required daily caloric intake. Eliminating gluten severely restricts one of the most bountiful components in a vegetarian's range of available options. For the gluten-free vegetarian, this loss will need to be compensated for by other food choices.

ALERT

By eliminating animal products from their diets, vegetarians are at a greater risk for nutrient deficiencies. These are generally well understood and compensated for by experienced vegetarians. Eliminating gluten may further jeopardize a vegetarian's ability to consume enough fiber, iron, and B vitamins for proper health. Talk to a nutritionist if you're a vegetarian adopting a gluten-free diet.

The other consideration vegetarians need to think about carefully is the use of wheat and gluten in vegetarian convenience products. Many meat substitutes, cheese substitutes, veggie dogs, veggie pepperoni, and mock turkey are all made with a combination of soy, vital wheat gluten, and other ingredients. Wheat gluten binds and gives texture to the finished product and is necessary in producing a realistic replica.

Textured vegetable protein (TVP) is often made with soy, but can also be made with wheat. Gluten-free vegetarians will need to spend extra time researching the ingredient list of products they buy to ensure the TVP used is safe for them to consume.

Taking supplements may be necessary if the vitamins and minerals necessary to maintain balanced nutrition are not being supplied by the foods eaten. Consult with your doctor or dietician to ensure that the proper supplements, in the proper quantities, are present in your diet.

Beginning a gluten-free diet can be a confusing time in your life. The long-term goal is improved health, but the short-term reality may be a time of adjustment, pain, and discomfort. Trying a few recipes, understanding what's in store for your body, and planning for the psychological and physiological symptoms of eliminating and detoxifying your body of gluten, will go a long way to helping you through this time of adjustment. Extending a different kind of restrictive diet, like vegetarianism, to gluten-free can cause similar problems. The difficulty you face may seem daunting at first. As your body heals, your health improves, and you become more comfortable with living gluten-free, the difficulty will also subside. Soon, the long-term goal of improved health and bodily healing will be realized, and there may even come a time when you wonder what all the fuss was about. Look forward to that time now and keep that goal in sight as you begin the journey of your gluten-free diet.

Explaining Your Diet to Others

Birthday parties, dinner parties, holidays, and gatherings all bring guests into your home. After all, living gluten-free won't, or shouldn't, halt your life. But guests may notice that the Caesar salad you serve contains no croutons, or the spaghetti and meat sauce doesn't come with garlic bread, and, polite as they may be, they may inquire about this. Don't shy away from these questions; instead, be prepared to explain your diet to anyone who asks.

There are several ways you can handle explaining your diet to others:

- You can assume that most people understand what a gluten-free diet is, and why it's necessary, and say very little.
- You can defuse any questions by being very up-front about your diet when you invite people over.
- You can wait until they begin asking questions about the food they are being served.

It is probably safe to assume that most people have heard of a gluten-free diet, but it's not a good idea to assume they understand all the reasons why you are adopting this lifestyle. In the case of biopsy-diagnosed celiac disease, they will need to understand that gluten is a toxin that damages your body and prevents it from functioning normally. Getting into the inner workings of the human gut is a conversation probably best left for some time other than at the dinner table. But a brief explanation of the condition followed by the statistics that approximately one in 133 people are living with the same condition may be all that's needed for your guests and friends to understand.

If you are hosting a child's birthday party, it might be best to say nothing about the diet to the guests. Tipping a child off that something is different about the food they are eating, regardless of whether it's gluten-free or not, can often elicit a negative response. Even changing brands of favorite foods can be enough to make a child wary about eating something. Don't say anything and see what happens. While even the best gluten-free baking will still taste different and have a slightly different texture from traditional baked goods, these differences will be minimal to the point of indistinguishable and will be overshadowed by the festivities, games, and gifts.

With adult guests, it might be fun to try "pulling a fast one" on them by serving them gluten-free food, including substitutes like bread and pasta, without telling them, just to see if they notice. Be fair by explaining to them afterward that you are on a gluten-free diet and they ate a gluten-free meal. They will probably be surprised, and delighted at the quality of the food. It might even dispel any misconceptions they may have had about gluten-free food. If you've done a good job in preparation, they won't be able to tell the difference.

CHAPTER 5

Beginning the Gluten-Free Lifestyle

Eliminating gluten from your diet can seem like a very over-whelming task. You may feel lost and miserable or like you will never be able to eat or enjoy food ever again. It's okay; everyone feels like that at first. Give yourself some time. Once you learn the ins and outs of the gluten-free diet, you will learn that you can still have your cake, and eat it too. Before you know it, you will be able to easily navigate your way around a grocery store or restaurant menu.

Out with the Old, In with the New: Restocking Your Pantry

When you first learn that your diet can no longer contain any gluten, you may think that simply *reducing* the amount of gluten-containing foods you eat will help you. In reality, however, removing all gluten from your diet at once is the best way to go. Simply reducing the amount of gluten you are consuming will still produce the same ill effects as a diet full of gluten. Eliminating all the food that contains gluten from your kitchen can seem like a huge undertaking at first, but just take it one step at a time.

To begin, eliminate any flours from your kitchen that are derived from wheat, oats, rye, or barley. That will include cake flour, pastry flour, self-rising flour, whole-wheat flour, and regular all-purpose flour. Be sure to carefully wash down any cupboards, drawers, or the pantry where you kept your flour. Flour can fall beside the container when you are scooping it, and you need to be sure to start with an area free of any gluten before restocking the pantry.

ALERT

To avoid getting sick from gluten residue, be sure to vacuum and scrub down all shelves, drawers, and cupboards where foods containing gluten were stored. Washing them with hot, soapy water, followed by wiping down with a clean, damp rag, should help remove all of the remaining gluten.

The next things that you need to remove from your kitchen are the baking ingredients that are derived from wheat, rye, barley, or oats. Since all of these items are derived from grains that contain gluten, they will need to be replaced as well. This would include wheat and oat bran, graham cracker crumbs, and chocolate cookie crumbs. While removing baking products, now would be an opportune time to remove the open containers of sugar, baking powder, baking soda, and salt. These products, although they do not contain gluten on their own, are most likely contaminated with gluten. Dipping a measuring cup or spoon into one ingredient after it has been used to measure flour will contaminate the second ingredient with gluten. For this reason, it is best to start your gluten-free kitchen with new, sealed containers.

After you remove the flours and baking supplies that contain gluten from the pantry, it is time to move on to the store-bought packaged items that obviously contain gluten. Those items include:

- Most crackers, cookies, cereal, and pasta, whether they are made with whole wheat, semolina, or durum-wheat
- Quick-to-prepare, packaged foods like noodles with sauce, instant oatmeal, gravy mixes, and many canned "cream of" soups

Getting Rid of Unsafe Foods

After going through your cupboards, pantry, fridge, and freezer and identifying all the food that contains gluten, you need to figure out what to do with all of it. Consider donating packages that are still closed and sealed to a local food bank or gifting them to friends or family. If packages are open, you can offer them to friends, family, or neighbors, but only do this with people that you know will be comfortable taking food from you. No one wants a neighbor, especially one they barely know, to come over and offer them an open box of cereal.

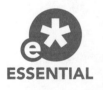

ESSENTIAL

There is a tremendous need for donations to food banks. An estimated 49 million Americans are living with food insecurity. Of those 49 million, almost 17 million are children and 5 million are seniors. According to the USDA Economic Research Service, Feeding America, more than 37 million people used a food bank for emergency food assistance in 2011.

Another possible solution for open cereal or pasta is donating it to a local day care, preschool, or school. Not for eating, but for crafting. Kids love to make pictures by gluing cereal or pasta to paper, or necklaces by stringing it onto a piece of yarn. Although not all child care facilities will be willing to accept an open package of food, some may be very appreciative.

Once you have exhausted all your resources in relocating your gluten-filled food by donating it, offering it to close friends and family, and restocking the crafting supplies of your local day care, the only thing left to do is to toss whatever remains in the garbage bin. Hopefully you will have found enough people willing to help you dispose of enough of your gluten-filled foods that you will not have to leave bags and bags of wasted food at the end of your driveway on garbage pickup day.

How to Read Labels at the Grocery Store

So far, all of the items that you have removed are obvious gluten-containing products, since they have been made with flour produced from wheat, rye, oats, or barley. But many other foods can contain hidden gluten. In order to know what to look for, you'll need to begin carefully reading all the labels on the food that you buy.

FACT

In the United States, as of fall 2012, the FDA has not finalized gluten-free standards. Since there is no regulation in place yet, some items that contain an unsafe amount of gluten are able to place a gluten-free label on the package. Always read the labels! You can find more information on the gluten-free labeling laws at *www.1in133.org*.

In 2006, the Food Allergen Labeling and Consumer Protection Act took effect. This act stipulates that if food products contain any of the top eight allergens, those ingredients must be clearly stated on the label. All products containing the following ingredients have to clearly state if any of those allergens are in that product, even if one of those items was "only" used to make one small part of the overall product:

1. Peanuts
2. Tree nuts
3. Eggs
4. Milk
5. Fish
6. Soy
7. Crustacean shellfish
8. Wheat

Although this law makes it easier to find wheat in products, it does not necessarily make it easier to find truly gluten-free items, since the labeling law doesn't cover ingredients containing rye, barley, and oats.

The Challenges with Barley and Oats

A product may have an allergy warning that says, "Contains wheat and soy," on the back of the package or, if one of the ingredients contains wheat, it will say something like "Natural Flavors (Wheat)" to let you know that an ingredient is derived from wheat. Remember, even if a label does not include a "contains wheat" warning, that does not make the product gluten-free, since rye and barley contain gluten and most commercially produced oats also contain trace amounts of gluten.

In addition to wheat, rye is also fairly easy to spot in an ingredient list because it is not used to make any other ingredients. Therefore it will simply be listed as "rye" on the label. Unfortunately, this is not the case with any of the other sources of gluten.

Barley is a difficult source to identify in processed foods. Besides being an obvious ingredient in beer, barley is also used to make other ingredients. For example, you can find it listed as barley malt, malt flavoring, malt vinegar, or even just malt.

ALERT

None of the oats available at your grocery store, whether quick-cook, old-fashioned, or steel-cut, is safe to consume if you are on a gluten-free diet. Also avoid the oats used in commonly available cookies, granola bars, cereals, and instant oatmeal. Never consume oats unless they clearly specify that they are "certified gluten-free."

Although commercially produced oats do not contain gluten, they remain unsafe for those that are on a gluten-free diet. Commercially produced oats may come into contact with wheat, barley, or rye while in the fields, during harvest, or while being transported, processed, or packaged. You can, however, purchase certified gluten-free oats. There are now specialized companies in Europe and North America that produce pure, uncontaminated oats that are grown on dedicated fields and are harvested and processed on dedicated equipment, like Bob's Red Mill and GF Harvest. Avoid any product that contains oats unless it is clearly specified that the oats are gluten-free.

Consult with your doctor prior to adding pure, uncontaminated oats to your gluten-free diet. In general, your celiac disease should be well controlled by your gluten-free diet, and you should no longer be experiencing any digestive problems before slowly introducing gluten-free oats into your diet.

"Hidden" Sources of Gluten to Avoid

The following is a list of ingredient terms to *avoid*. Some are easy to notice—for instance, if you saw "wheat bran extract," you would avoid it because of the word "wheat." Others are not so obvious, so it's good to try to commit them to memory, or keep this list handy as you shop:

- Barley
- Couscous (made from wheat)
- Farina (made from wheat)
- Flour varieties: spelt, triticale, durum, einkorn, emmer, farina, semolina, Kamut, and bulgur (These are sometimes listed as "wheat" on labels. Although they contain less gluten than wheat, they do still contain gluten and should be omitted from your diet.)
- Groats
- Hordeum vulgare (barley)
- Malt (made from barley)
- Malt extract
- Malt syrup
- Malt flavoring
- Malt vinegar
- Maltose
- Pasta (made from wheat unless otherwise indicated)
- Pearl barley
- Rice malt
- Rye
- Secale cereale (rye)
- Seitan (made from wheat gluten and commonly used in vegetarian meals)
- Sprouted barley

- Triticale (cross between wheat and rye)
- Triticum spelta (spelt, a form of wheat)
- Triticum vulgare (wheat)
- Oat
- Wheat
- Wheat flour/bread flour/bleached flour
- Wheat germ oil or extract (could be cross contaminated)
- Wheat or barley grass (could be cross contaminated)
- Wheat protein/hydrolyzed wheat protein
- Wheat starch/hydrolyzed wheat starch

If any of the following terms are included in the ingredient list on a label, it means that the product *may* contain gluten, but it depends on what the product is derived from. It could be derived from a grain that contains gluten, or it could be derived from soy, corn, or other gluten-free grains. If you are unsure of the origin of an ingredient, it is best to call the manufacturer to find out if the product is gluten-free.

- Vegetable protein/hydrolyzed vegetable protein (can come from wheat, corn, or soy)
- Modified starch/modified food starch (can come from several sources, including wheat)
- Natural flavor/natural flavoring (can come from barley)
- Artificial flavor/artificial flavoring (can come from barley)
- Modified food starch
- Hydrolyzed plant protein/HPP
- Hydrolyzed vegetable protein/HVP
- Seasonings
- Fillers and binders
- Flavorings
- Vegetable starch
- Dextrin and maltodextrin (In the United States, maltodextrin is usually made from rice, corn, or potato. In Europe, maltodextrin is frequently made from wheat.)

Foods That Are Safe to Eat

Listed below are a few foods and ingredients that you may be unsure about, but they *are safe* to consume on a gluten-free diet.

- **Alcoholic beverages (most):** All distilled liquors are safe to drink, even if the grains that are fermented to produce the alcohol contain gluten. The gluten is not carried over during the distilling process, and the end result contains no gluten. Champagne, brandy, vodka, scotch, and rum are all safe to drink if you are on a gluten-free diet, even if they are derived from wheat, rye, or barley. Be sure to read labels on premade drink mixes, as they may contain barley malt. Liqueurs, including Baileys Irish Cream, are gluten-free. The distilling process for beer, however, is different from that of liquor, and beers that are made using wheat, rye, or barley still contain gluten after they are processed. There are gluten-free beers available that are made from grains like sorghum, rice, or buckwheat.

ALERT

Most bottled red and white wines are gluten-free; however, a few old wineries still use oak barrels that are sealed with a paste made from wheat. It is best to research the winery to find out if a particular wine is completely gluten-free.

- **Beans:** All beans are gluten-free, including adzuki, black beans, chickpea, kidney, lentils, and romano. You still have to read the labels on beans that have been processed, either into baked beans or canned beans, to ensure that no ingredients that have been added contain gluten.
- **Buckwheat:** Despite having "wheat" in its name, buckwheat is actually safe to eat for those on a gluten-free diet. Buckwheat is a fruit, resembling the berry of a wheat plant, from the Polygonaceae family. The Polygonaceae family of plants also includes rhubarb and sorrel, neither of which contain gluten.
- **Distilled vinegar:** Despite controversy in the past over vinegar, rest assured that it is gluten-free. Vinegar can be made using wheat, corn,

potatoes, or wood. The distilling process, in a manner similar to liquor, removes the gluten from the product, making it safe for those eating a gluten-free diet. Safe vinegars include white vinegar, red or white wine vinegar, balsamic vinegar, apple cider vinegar, sherry vinegar, and rice wine vinegar.

QUESTION

Does malt vinegar contain gluten?
The only vinegar that remains controversial is malt vinegar. Some argue that, after fermenting and production, only a trace amount of gluten exists. Others insist it is unsafe because it is derived from barley in the first place. Check with your doctor to see what he or she advises.

- **Glucose syrup, Maltodextrin, Dextrose, and Monosodium Glutamate (MSG):** Although all of these ingredients are derived from wheat or barley, they have all undergone a breaking-down process during production, at which time the gluten has been removed, making it safe for people on a gluten-free diet to consume.
- **Glutinous Rice Flour:** Also called sweet rice flour, glutinous rice flour does not contain any gluten. Instead, it is made from short-grained, sticky rice.

Check Everything!

You might find gluten in still *more* places while you're shopping, so it's important to read every label. Here is a list of some foods, which you probably wouldn't think of checking, that *may* contain gluten:

- Lunch meats/sausages
- Meat substitutes
- Barbecue sauce/condiments
- Nuts/dried fruit
- Corn chips/potato chips
- Licorice/candy/chocolate
- Ice cream/yogurt
- Blended tea/herbal tea

- Makeup/creams and lotions
- Toothpaste
- Medication/vitamins

If you have questions about whether a product contains gluten, contact the manufacturer, or ask your health care provider.

Making Sense of Gluten-Free Flours and Starches

When you initially begin your gluten-free journey, you might wonder how you can ever eat breads, cookies, or pizza again without having flour in your life. Do not despair; you only have to eliminate the flours made from wheat, rye, and barley. Your world is now going to open up to a large bouquet of gluten-free flours, some that you may have never heard of before.

Unlike wheat flour, none of the gluten-free flours or starches can be used in a stand-alone manner when baking. Gluten-free baking that yields the best results will require combinations of flours and starches. Baking cookies with just rice flour will result in a very crumbly cookie. Baking a cake with only oat flour will result in a heavy cake that falls in the middle. But by using a combination of different gluten-free flours and starches, as well as some xanthan or guar gum, you will be able to replicate nearly any of your favorite gluten-filled baked goods.

Each of the gluten-free flours and starches has their own distinct texture and flavor, and each of the flours and starches will bring their own characteristics to the blend. It may take some experimenting to find a mix that works best and produces the desired results in the recipes you're trying. Following are some of the most often used and readily available flours and starches used in gluten-free baking.

Grains

- **Rice flour:** Rice flour is the most commonly used flour in gluten-free baking, both homemade and commercially produced. Rice flour is made by milling the grains of rice into a fine powder. When buying rice flour, look for the word "superfine" on the package as this will eliminate a gritty texture in finished baked goods.

- White rice flour, which has a pretty bland flavor, is used to add lightness and texture to gluten-free goods.
- Brown rice flour, which has a nuttier flavor, adds nutrients and fiber. Brown rice has over three times more fiber than white rice.
- Sweet rice flour (also called glutinous rice flour, but containing no gluten) is milled from a short grain, sticky rice and has higher starch content than white or brown rice flour. It is used to impart a slightly chewy texture to baked goods. It is also often used as a thickener for sauces.
- **Cornstarch:** Cornstarch is one of the most common gluten-free starches. It's most often used to thicken gravies and sauces, but it also works well to add tenderness to gluten-free baking. Cornstarch is one of the main ingredients in shortbread cookies because it helps to produce a crumbly, tender-textured cookie. Many batter recipes use cornstarch because of the light, crisp crust that it forms after frying. Cornstarch is a good substitute for potato starch and arrowroot flour.

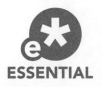

ESSENTIAL

When using cornstarch as a thickener in sauces, mix the cornstarch with a small amount of cold water before adding it to the heated sauce to thicken. If you add it directly to heated sauce, the cornstarch will clump together and make the sauce lumpy. Cornstarch is called "corn flour" in Europe.

- **Corn flour:** Not to be confused with cornstarch, corn flour is high in fiber and has a slight nutty flavor. Masa harina, a form of corn flour, is milled from whole corn that has been soaked in limewater. Masa harina is used to make corn tortillas and tamale dough. Corn flour can also be used to replace a portion of cornmeal in a recipe to give it a lighter, less crumbly texture.
- **Cornmeal:** Cornmeal is one of the main ingredients in corn bread. It is more coarsely ground than corn flour. Cornmeal comes in yellow, white, or blue varieties, and in fine, medium, or course grinds. Corn-

meal is usually mixed with corn flour or other flours making up, in general, no more than 25 percent of the flour blend. There are exceptions to this rule, though, since some corn bread recipes call for only cornmeal. Selecting the correct grind of cornmeal for the recipe is important. If the grind is too coarse, food may have a gritty texture to it. Coarse cornmeal makes a wonderful breading, and finer grinds make great corn bread, pancakes, and polenta.

- **Amaranth flour:** Although this ancient grain of the Aztecs can be ground into flour that is sweet with a slightly nutty flavor, it is to be used sparingly, no more than 10–20 percent of your flour blend. Amaranth works best in recipes that do not contain a lot of liquid. It browns quickly and forms a thicker crust, and it also performs best in recipes that use brown rice syrup or maple syrup as the sweetener.

- **Millet flour:** Millet is considered one of the oldest grains consumed by humans. Millet is a high-protein, high-nutrient flour that is easily digested. Millet flour works great in breads, flat breads, pizza, and other items containing yeast. It can be used up to 25 percent in a flour blend, and it imparts a slight yellow color and nutty flavor to baked goods. Millet flour needs to be stored in an airtight container in the refrigerator or freezer to keep it from going rancid and having a bitter taste.

- **Sorghum flour:** Sorghum is a high-protein, high-fiber flour that actually has a slight wheat-like flavor. You can also find it on the shelves under the name milo or jowar flour. Because of the flour's darker color, most bakers suggest that sorghum not be used in baked goods that should look white. Sorghum can be used up to 30 percent in a flour blend, and is great for breads, muffins, cookies, and pancakes. Sorghum flour should be stored in an airtight container or in the refrigerator to extend its shelf life.

- **Teff flour:** Teff is an ancient grain that has been an important food source in Ethiopia for thousands of years. Teff flour, which is high in protein, calcium, and fiber, can come in light or dark varieties and imparts a mild, nutty flavor to baked goods. Add only a small amount of teff flour to baked goods to improve the nutritional value. Teff flour works well in cookies, cakes, quick breads, waffles, and pancakes. It is best to refrigerate teff flour to increase its shelf life.

- **Oats and oat flour:** Pure, uncontaminated, certified gluten-free oats and oat flour are great to use in your gluten-free baking. High in fiber, protein, and nutrition, oats add taste and texture to baked goods. You can use oats or oat flour in breads, cookies, cakes, muffins, and pancakes. Certified gluten-free oats also make great granola and granola bars. Be sure to talk to your doctor before adding oats, or oat flour, to your diet. Bakers recommended that oat flour not exceed 30 percent of your flour blend.

Tuber and Root Starches

- **Arrowroot flour:** Arrowroot flour can be used in place of cornstarch in recipes. It is great to use as a batter coating for fish, chicken, and vegetables. Arrowroot flour adds good body and texture to gluten-free baked goods, and it also works well as a thickener for sauces. It is pleasant-tasting and a versatile flour that works great for breads and bagels. Bakers suggest that you can use up to 25 percent arrowroot flour in your flour blend.

FACT

Arrowroot flour is made from the thick stem of the Bermuda arrow-root plant. This plant is native to the West Indies and Central America. If used as a thickener, in a sauce, it is important to not overcook it. If arrowroot flour is overcooked, the sauce will become runny again.

- **Potato starch:** Different from potato flour, potato starch is made from the starch of dehydrated potatoes. It has no protein or fat, and is often used to help lighten a flour blend, but does not usually make up more than 33 percent of the flour blend. Potato starch can be substituted for cornstarch one-for-one.
- **Potato flour:** Not to be confused with potato starch, potato flour is made by grinding the whole dried potato into flour. It is high in fiber and protein. Adding 2 to 4 tablespoons to a bread, homemade pasta, or pizza crust recipe will give the goods a nice chewy texture. You do

not want to use too much potato flour in a recipe, or the texture will be gummy instead of chewy.

- **Tapioca starch:** Tapioca starch and tapioca flour are the same thing; it could be labeled in stores under either name. Tapioca starch is derived from the cassava plant and is well tolerated by most people, even those who have multiple food allergies. It should be used as part of a flour blend, but no more than 20 percent. If more than 20 percent of your flour blend is tapioca starch, you will end up with a gummy texture to your baked goods. Tapioca starch helps give baked goods a chewy texture, and also increases the browning capacities of baked goods. It is a great choice for breads, pasta, and tortillas, and can be used as a thickener in gravies and sauces.

Beans and Legumes

Dried beans can be ground into flour as well. These include garbanzo (chickpea), soy, romano, fava, navy, pinto, red, or white beans. Bean flours are high in protein and fiber, and help baked goods retain moisture and add desirable texture. Sometimes garbanzo bean flour is blended with fava bean flour, creating "Garfava flour."

Bakers suggest that you use no more than 25 percent of bean flour in your flour blend. Not everyone likes the flavor of bean flours, and some people experience non-gluten-related digestive distress from the flours, so take that into account before using it. Bean flours work great in breads and pizza and especially well in spice cakes.

Nut Flours

- **Almond flour:** Almond flour or almond meal is created by grinding blanched almonds. Almond meal is high in protein and healthy fats. By adding almond flour to your gluten-free baked goods, you are going to be adding moisture, flavor, and texture and improving the nutritional value of your cakes, cookies, and cupcakes. You can make your own almond flour by grinding blanched almonds in a coffee grinder, but be careful, almond flour can become almond butter very quickly. Because of the high protein value of almond flour, you can use it as a replacement for dry milk powder when baking for the lactose intolerant. Almond flour can also be used to makes a fantastic breading for chicken and fish, or as a substitute for oats in oatmeal cookies. Because of the high fat content of almond flour, it is best to store it in the fridge in an airtight container.

- **Chestnut flour:** Chestnut flour is made from ground whole chestnuts and can be used in gluten-free baking. Popular in rich Italian and French pastries, chestnut flour gives the baked goods a sweet, nutty flavor while increasing the fiber. Chestnut flour, however, is very low in protein and works best when paired with high-protein flours, like bean, amaranth, or soy, to ensure that the baked goods will not be crumbly. Do not use more than 20 percent chestnut flour in your flour blend—too much will give the flour a strong, earthy taste that can be unpleasant.

- **Coconut flour:** This high-fiber, low-carbohydrate flour, which has a sweet coconut smell, has become quite popular. Although it is possible to bake using just coconut flour, it is usually used in small quantities, about 15 percent of your flour blend. Coconut flour is 60 percent fiber, but fairly high in fat. If you use too much coconut flour in your recipe, your baked goods can turn out very dense. If you increase the amount of coconut flour in your recipe, you should also increase the amount of eggs or liquids in your recipe. Coconut flour absorbs nearly four times the amount of liquid as wheat flour.

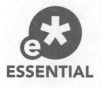

ESSENTIAL

Coconut flour has more than twice the amount of dietary fiber compared to wheat bran. The high amount of dietary fiber in coconut flour helps to stabilize blood sugar levels by slowing down the release of glucose. Glucose is transported to the cells where it is transformed into energy. A slower rate of glucose release, into the body, results in a more moderate need for insulin.

Seed Flours

- **Quinoa:** Although quinoa is an ancient grain, it has only recently become very popular. It is considered a complete protein, meaning that it has an adequate amount of all nine of the essential amino acids necessary in the human diet. Because of its high protein content, quinoa, which is also easy to digest, has been labeled a "superfood." It can be used as a whole seed, as flakes, or ground into a flour. Quinoa, which is also high in fiber, calcium, and protein, can be used to increase the nutritional value of your flour blend. Quinoa flour can make up to 25 percent of your flour blend, but adding too much can give your baked goods a strong, bitter flavor. Quinoa flakes can be used to replace oats in recipes for cookies, breads, cakes, and granola.

- **Flaxseed meal:** Ground flaxseed is something that you may have stocked in your kitchens before going gluten-free. That's because, among a multitude of other health benefits, flaxseed helps to lower cholesterol. Flax is high in fiber and omega-3 fatty acids, but the nutrients—protected inside the seed by its little hard shell—are only released and available to be absorbed by the body when it is ground. Try adding a few tablespoons to your bread or pancake recipe to increase the nutritional value. Ground flax also adds stability and texture to gluten-free baked breads. You can grind whole flaxseeds into flaxseed meal using a coffee grinder. Ground flaxseed should be stored in the fridge or freezer, since the high fat content can cause it to go rancid quickly.

FACT

You can use ground flaxseed as an egg substitute when baking muffins, cakes, and breads. Mix one tablespoon of ground flaxseed with three tablespoons of hot water, stir, and allow the mixture to stand for ten minutes before using. This amount replaces one egg.

All-Purpose Gluten-Free Flour Blends

There are some premade "all-purpose" gluten-free flour mixes available at some supermarkets nowadays. These usually work best in baked goods like cookies and muffins—items that would not require a lot of gluten even if baked with traditional flour. Baking breads and chewy pizza crusts is possible with gluten-free flours, but it will require more modifications to a recipe than just mixing and switching flours and adding the gum (guar or xanthan) of your choice. With breads, you usually need to add more liquids, sometimes in the form of an extra egg or egg white, and a little extra leavening. This can be achieved by adding more egg whites or by adding apple cider vinegar and some baking soda.

It's also possible to mix an "all-purpose" gluten-free flour blend by whisking together 4 cups of brown rice flour, $1^1/_3$ cups of potato starch (not potato flour), and $^2/_3$ cup of tapioca starch/flour. This all-purpose flour blend is a great starting point when learning to bake gluten-free. You still have to add either xanthan or guar gum to this mix, with the amount being determined by what you are baking. If you are using a commercially manufactured gluten-free flour blend, be sure to read the label to see if either xanthan or guar gums have already been added.

Keeping It All Together: Gums

Gluten is the protein that binds flour and other ingredients together. It allows dough to stretch and holds bubbles that leavening agents have formed in the dough. When you remove gluten, breads fall, cookies crumble, and cakes go flat. Some structure can be created in your baked goods from eggs and the flours themselves, but to help recreate the texture and mouth-feel of gluten-filled baked goods, you need to use other additives. Xanthan gum and guar gum are the two most commonly used additives. They are used to bind, emulsify, and thicken gluten-free ingredients.

Xanthan Gum

Xanthan gum is the most commonly used gluten substitute in gluten-free baking. It is made by fermenting sugars (glucose, sucrose, or lactose) with a microbial called *Xanthomonas campestris*. Xanthan gum should be used sparingly in gluten-free baking. Too much xanthan gum will produce a dense, gummy, sometimes slimy, product. Xanthan gum is usually preferred over guar gum, even though it costs more, because it is easier to digest. While some xanthan gums are produced by fermenting a corn sugar, the Bob's Red Mill brand states that its xanthan gum is produced by feeding micro-organisms "a glucose solution that is derived from wheat starch." Not to worry though, their xanthan gum is still gluten-free. "Gluten is found in the protein part of the wheat kernel and no gluten is contained in the solution of glucose," the Bob's Red Mill marketing information explains. "Additionally, after the bacteria has [*sic*] eaten the glucose, there is no wheat to be found in the outer coating that it produces, which is what makes up xanthan gum."

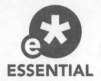

Guar Gum

Guar gum is a natural thickener, made by grinding a bean-like seed from the guar plant, or Indian tree, into a fine powder. Until 1990, guar gum was a major component of nonprescription weight-loss pills. The high fiber content of guar gum would cause the user to feel fuller longer. Guar gum became a problem when, due to the large amounts being consumed, people began developing digestive issues. Subsequently, it was banned from use in nonprescription pills by the FDA. Some people find that due to the high fiber content of guar gum, it can cause digestive problems even when used in small amounts for gluten-free baking. Measure carefully when using guar gum; using too much will result in a dense, stringy texture in your baked products.

Which Gum to Use

Figure out which gum will work best for your baking by determining a few things. First, consider the cost—guar gum costs nearly half as much as xanthan gum. However, if you are unable to digest any baked goods that use guar gum, xanthan gum may be the better gum for you to use.

The amount of xanthan or guar gum needed in a recipe varies by the type of recipe. Cookies and muffins will require quite a bit less gum than bread dough. This is similar to conventional baking where it is important to not over-stir muffin batter, keeping the gluten development to a minimum. Bread dough, on the other hand, has to be kneaded until the gluten has fully developed and the dough is elastic. Choosing an ingredient to replace gluten, and the amount to use, must be made with similar considerations in mind.

The following is a guideline for how much xanthan gum to add to a recipe. You'll probably need to experiment a few times to get the desired result for the recipe you're using.

- Cookies: ¼ teaspoon per cup of gluten-free flour
- Cakes and pancakes: ½ teaspoon per cup of gluten-free flour
- Muffins and quick breads: ¾ teaspoon per cup of gluten-free flour
- Breads: 1 to 1½ teaspoons per cup of gluten-free flour
- Pizza dough: 2 teaspoons per cup of gluten-free flour

To substitute xanthan gum with guar gum, the common recommendation is to multiply the amount of xanthan gum by 1.5 and use that amount. As an example, if a recipe calls for 1 teaspoon of xanthan gum, you can substitute 1½ teaspoons of guar gum.

Gum Substitutes

Some people on a gluten-free diet find that xanthan gum and guar gum give them nongluten digestive issues, such as gas and bloating. Some bakers who decide to not use either gum have been successful in using ground flaxseed and ground chia seeds in their place. If a recipe calls for two teaspoons of xanthan gum, use 1 teaspoon of ground flaxseed and 1 teaspoon of ground chia seed mixed with 4 teaspoons of boiling water. Stir the mixture and let it sit for 10 minutes to create a gelatinous slurry before adding this to your batter or dough.

Keep in mind that adding too much ground chia seed to your bread may cause your bread to become gummy. For breads, begin with 1 to 2 teaspoons of ground chia seeds and 2 tablespoons of ground flaxseed mixed with 5 tablespoons of boiling water. Using ground flax and chia seed will not give you the same mouth-feel as using xanthan or guar gum would, but it will reduce the amount of crumbliness that your baked goods would have without adding anything.

ALERT

If you do not use xanthan gum or guar gum in your gluten-free baking, increasing the protein content in your dough may also help produce the desired results. Protein content can be increased by using an extra egg, dry milk powder, or high-protein flours like sorghum, bean flours, or teff.

Finding Gluten in Your Medicine Cabinet and Makeup Bag

Once you've cleaned out some gluten-containing foods from your pantry, it's time to check your medicine cabinet and your makeup bag. Manufacturers sometimes use wheat, rye, barley, or oat products in lipstick, shampoo, toothpaste, lotions, supplements, and medication.

Start by checking any lipstick or lip balm products, since cosmetics, lotions, or creams that are applied close to your mouth can easily be ingested. If you are on a gluten-free diet and your lipstick contains gluten, you could still be ingesting it and could be experiencing the harmful effects that gluten can have on your body.

Checking your makeup bag can be tricky as there are no labeling laws regarding gluten in cosmetic products. Since some sub-ingredients may have been derived from a gluten-containing product, it is best to call the manufacturer to confirm whether the products you are using are gluten-free. COVERGIRL is one major cosmetics company that understands this concern and wants their customers to be well informed. When contacted about their products, they quickly responded:

"We know Celiac is a serious disease, so we want to give you clear information regarding the use of our beauty care products. If wheat and/or gluten aren't directly added to a product by us, these ingredients won't be listed on our packages. Like many companies, we often purchase the scents for fragranced products from outside suppliers, and the components of these substances are proprietary information belonging to those companies. Therefore it's possible that a very small amount (generally parts per million) of gluten may be present.

The same process is true of many cosmetic companies, so see if your favorite brand will disclose the ingredients that they do control.

You can find gluten-free cosmetic companies, dedicated to producing a complete line of products for celiac and gluten-sensitive customers. To ensure the contents of your makeup bag is 100 percent gluten-free, stick with companies like Afterglow Cosmetics, Ecco Bella, Red Apple Lipstick, Lavera Naturkosmetik, and NARS Cosmetics. There are others, so feel free to shop around, ask questions, and see what you can find. Start with retailers that carry organic and all-natural beauty products. Companies that are already conscientious about the ingredients in their products, for other reasons, are more likely to also carry products that do not contain gluten.

Hair care products and lotions are another potential source of gluten that need to be checked. Since shampoo and conditioner wash down your face, and hairspray is sprayed into the air, you could accidentally ingest any gluten that they contain. Body lotions are another potential source. Even if you apply the lotion far from your mouth, you will be applying it with your hands where it could linger until you touch your face, or eat something, transferring the gluten to your mouth.

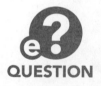

QUESTION

Can gluten be absorbed through the skin?
Although it has been proven that gluten molecules are too large to be absorbed through the skin, many people claim they feel the effects of gluten if they apply cosmetics and other personal products that contain gluten. Regardless of this debate, the reality is that products used on your body could come into contact with your lips or mouth, and you could end up ingesting gluten. It's best to avoid that problem by eliminating all potential sources, no matter how remote they may seem.

Watch for the following gluten-containing ingredients when you are trying to determine if a product contains gluten:

- Avena sativa
- Barley extract
- Barley solids

- Hydrolyzed wheat protein
- Hydrolyzed wheat starch
- Hydrolyzed wheat gluten
- Hordeum vulgare
- Amino peptide complex
- Triticum vulgare
- Oat bran
- Oat flour
- Oat extract
- Oat protein
- Phytosphingosine extract
- Vitamin E derived from wheat germ
- Wheat germ oil
- Wheat germ extract
- Wheat germ glycerides

If the product contains any of these names, it should be considered NOT safe for those living gluten-free.

ALERT

The dentist's office is often overlooked as a potential source of gluten. Some latex gloves contain a powder—a drying agent to assist in glove removal—that may contain gluten. Fluoride and polish used in tooth cleaning may also contain gluten. Call a few days before your appointment to address these concerns and request a gluten-free appointment.

Read the labels on supplements, over-the-counter medication, and prescription drugs very carefully. Currently, there are no laws requiring that allergens be clearly labeled on these products. If you are unsure if your medication is gluten-free, talk to your doctor or pharmacist and get answers. Don't overlook this potential source; ingesting gluten from your medication will be just as harmful as eating a gluten-filled cookie.

Check the list of gluten-free medications at *www.glutenfreedrugs.com*. This website is a helpful resource maintained by pharmacists at Nationwide Children's Hospital in Columbus, Ohio.

CHAPTER 6

Your Gluten-Free Kitchen

Once you start your gluten-free diet, you may be spending more time in the kitchen than you used to. The extra care and attention that is required to maintain a gluten-free diet will require you to prepare more of your meals and snacks at home, in your gluten-free kitchen. Take advantage of this opportunity to make fresh, healthy meals using your decontaminated pantry and equipment.

Kitchen Tools: What to Clean and What to Replace

Gluten can lurk everywhere in a kitchen, but taking a careful walk-through and inspecting everything will help you identify the equipment that you need to clean or replace to make your kitchen gluten-free. Although most of your kitchen equipment and tools are still safe to use when you are preparing gluten-free foods, there are a few items that you should consider replacing outright.

Getting rid of some of your kitchen equipment may seem like a horrible waste, but all is not lost. While you are purging the dangerous items, you may find this a great time to add to the safe kitchen equipment that you already have. After seeing how expensive store-bought gluten-free food can be, you may decide to do more cooking and baking than you ever did before going gluten-free. Don't fear this process, it's a great adventure and every adventure needs to be properly outfitted.

Toaster

Start by replacing your toaster. The toaster is one of the few kitchen items that you cannot easily clean. The design of even the best toasters leaves many nooks, crannies, and areas that are difficult to reach to properly clean. Toast produces so many crumbs that, no matter how well you try to clean them, toasters that have been used for regular breads will have gluten in them. Again, since the chance of cross-contamination is extremely high, it is best to not use a toaster that has been used for wheat-based breads—not for gluten-free breads, anyway. If you insist on continuing to use the same toaster, one way to safely do so is by using toaster safe bags. ToastIt Toaster Bags (*www.amazon.com/dp/B0012XGM92*) are heatproof, reusable bags that hold your bread when placing it in the toaster. These bags will keep the crumbs of wheat-based bread from coming into contact with your healthy, delicious, safe, gluten-free bread.

FACT

ToastIt Toaster Bags are made from Teflon coated fabric and are heat resistant up to 500°F. They are nonstick and can simply be wiped out or washed and left to air-dry. ToastIt Toaster Bags can be reused up to 50 times before they need replacing.

Bowls, Pots, and Pans

Scrutinize all your plastic mixing bowls and nonstick frying pans. Both of these items can easily get scratched over time and those scratches can trap and hold gluten in them. Even after a good, thorough scrubbing, the dents, divots, dings, and damage done to a bowl or pan over the course of its working life can accumulate tiny particles of gluten. Buying a new frying pan and metal or ceramic mixing bowls will help to eliminate the risk of gluten contamination. Even if you maintain a shared kitchen (a kitchen that produces both gluten and gluten-free items), bowls made from these materials are much easier to properly clean. You can remove the gluten proteins from these smooth surfaces with a good scrubbing, using hot water and soap.

Cutting Boards

Replace your cutting board when you switch your kitchen to gluten-free. Or, keep an extra dedicated gluten-free board on hand. Many times, bread is sliced on a cutting board and like plastic bowls, the scratches and nicks in the cutting board work perfectly to trap gluten. If you have a shared kitchen, be sure to clearly label which cutting board is to be used for gluten-free products only.

ALERT

It is very easy to accidentally mix up cutting boards. Buying colored cutting boards can help you remember which cutting board is being used for gluten-free food. Designate one color for gluten-free foods, and the other for foods that contain gluten.

Colanders

When you use a colander to drain wheat-based pasta, the high amount of starch in the pasta can leave starchy residue on the colander, which can remain even if it is thoroughly washed. It is nearly impossible to make sure that all the little holes in the colander are completely clear of gluten. The next time it is used to drain gluten-free pasta, it will become contaminated with gluten from this residue. Purchase a new one and clearly label it to be used for gluten-free food only.

Wooden Utensils

Wooden utensils, such as salad servers and stirring spoons, should be replaced. In addition to scratches, the wood has a porous surface that may trap gluten the same way that a scratched plastic bowl can.

ESSENTIAL

Even though more prepackaged gluten-free foods are becoming readily available, they are often higher in calories and lower in nutrients than homemade foods. Commercial producers often increase the amount of sugar and fat in store-bought gluten-free foods to help improve the flavor. This is another reason to put on your apron and get cooking.

Baking Equipment

Learning how to bake your favorite foods—without gluten—early in your journey will help ensure you don't feel deprived of anything.

Baking Pans

Light-colored, commercial-grade baking pans are one great investment for any kitchen. A rectangular baking pan with low edges is one of the most important and often used pans in a kitchen. These pans are great for baking cookies or squares and can be used for oven-roasting meat or vegetables. Overall, they are versatile and make great, multipurpose kitchen items to have on hand. The size of the baking pan that you need will depend on the portion size—how many people you are baking for—and how large your oven is.

FACT

You will want to make sure any pan you buy will leave a few inches of space between the outside of the pan itself and your oven wall. This will ensure that the air can still circulate in your oven, allowing your food to bake evenly. If the baking pan reaches all the way to the oven walls, the oven temperature will increase by as much as 50°F, causing your food to bake too quickly, or even to burn.

Investing in a heavier gauge, properly sized baking sheet will ensure that you get better results all the time. Cheaper pans tend to warp when they get hot, and nonstick pans tend to scratch and peel over time. A good aluminium baking pan is a "must" if you intend to do a lot of baking.

Here's another tip: Lining your baking pan with parchment paper is another way to get great results every time you bake. Greasing your cookie sheets won't provide enough protection from sticking when baking gluten-free. Cookies will tend to stick and then crumble when you try to remove them from the pan. When baking pans are lined with parchment paper, cookies release easily and you also have a much easier time cleaning your pans after baking.

Stand Mixers

Stand mixers are one of the most useful kitchen appliances for baking gluten-free. Having one is not a necessity, nor is buying one a small expense, but many people find it to be a great addition to a gluten-free kitchen. If you were not a baker prior to starting a gluten-free diet, you may want to consider becoming one now.

A stand mixer can be used for mixing cookies, cakes, bread, and pizza dough, and it can also be used for other things like mixing the ingredients for meatloaf, making mashed potatoes, and shredding cooked chicken. If you can envision yourself baking and cooking for years to come, then a stand mixer is a great investment. Heavy-duty hand mixers are good and can be used effectively, yet they have a lot less power than a stand mixer. If you expect to use a mixer multiple times a week—sometimes multiple times a day—a stand mixer's motor will last a lot longer than a hand-held mixer. Because a stand mixer's bowl is made of stainless steel or glass, it is possible to share the mixer with both gluten-free and wheat-based dough, as long as it is carefully cleaned in between uses.

Kitchen Equipment Safety for All!

Now that you are spending more time in the contaminant-free kitchen, preparing delicious, safe food on dedicated—in some cases new—kitchen equipment, it's time to remind yourself of general safety tips for cooking. Here are a few essentials to keep in mind while working in the kitchen.

- Always use the proper equipment with the proper appliance. If a baking dish is not clearly labeled as microwave safe, for example, don't use it in the microwave. Likewise, a casserole dish may be safe to use in the oven, but may not be safely used on a stovetop. Improper use of kitchen equipment can result in serious injuries to yourself or loved ones, not to mention damage to your kitchen. Always read the warnings that come with your kitchen equipment.
- Be sure that all pot handles on the stovetop and counter are turned in and not sticking out past the countertop. This will help ensure that you do not accidentally hook on to them and that no small children can pull them off the counter.
- Wear properly fitted clothing when working in the kitchen. Long, draping sleeves can hook on to things, or get too close to hot elements.
- Always be extra careful with sharp objects, such as knives and vegetable peelers. Always keep the blade facing down and cut away from yourself. Even lids that have been removed from cans can have a very sharp edge, so be careful when removing, cleaning, and discarding them. When storing knives in a drawer, make sure that they have some sort of cover for the blades so that you do not accidentally cut yourself when you reach in to remove the knife. If the knives are stored on a magnetic strip, make sure that the magnet is strong enough to hold the knife securely, and that the magnetic strip is securely fastened to the wall.
- Always use proper oven mitts when removing items from the oven. Using a cloth or dishtowel will not properly protect you from the hot pans and racks.
- Steam can burn you. Even though you may not see any dangerous red elements or other warning signs, this nearly-invisible danger is very real. When removing a lid from a boiling pot, stand back and carefully remove the lid so that the steam will not touch you. If you stand with your face over the pot, or remove the lid so that the steam releases onto your arm, you can badly burn yourself.
- Always have a fire extinguisher nearby. One-third of all house fires begin in the kitchen, so it is better to be safer rather than sorry. Grease fires are extremely common in kitchens and can start in a matter of minutes. Never throw water on a fire that involves grease, as it will

only spread the fire. Instead, sprinkle the fire with baking soda or use a proper fire extinguisher to put the fire out.

QUESTION

What kind of fire extinguisher is best to have in the kitchen?
A "Class B" fire extinguisher or a general purpose extinguisher suitable for Class A, B, and C fires is best for kitchens. These extinguishers contain fire-suppressant chemicals suitable for fires involving grease and oil. Class A extinguishers contain only water, which will not extinguish oil or grease fires and may even cause the fire to spread further.

- Any time you are working with oil, use a cooking thermometer to watch the temperature. It doesn't matter how much oil there is in a pan, if it gets too hot it can start a fire, which can quickly get out of control. If oil does get too hot, turn off the heating element, place a lid on the pot, and leave the oil to cool down slowly. If you are deep-frying, never move a pot of hot oil from one location to another. Any spills can cause serious burns. If a small fire should occur, pour baking soda on the fire and cover the pot with a tight fitting lid. Never move a pot that is on fire, as you can cause much more damage by trying to move it. *Never leave heating oil unattended.*

- If you are using a stand mixer, food processor, or a blender, always make sure that the machine is turned off before scraping down the sides of the container. Getting your fingers or cooking utensils caught in a moving mixer or blender could cause serious personal injury.

- It is great to have children help you in the kitchen, but be clear in your instructions to them, and keep careful watch over them. Children can easily misunderstand instructions and, if left unattended even for a moment, could badly injure themselves.

- Always be sure that the cords for your electric appliances are not broken or cracked, and that they are kept away from water at all times. A crack in the plastic coating on the cords makes them dangerous to operate and, if cords are exposed to water, you run the risk of getting a serious electric shock.

Spicing Up Your Spice Rack

Adding herbs and spices to your culinary creations is one of the best and easiest ways to liven up your food as you transition to gluten-free cooking. It's best to use fresh ingredients, but that's not always possible, so having a stable of dried ingredients is essential. Using dried herbs and spices is extremely convenient as well. But do you need to worry about gluten hiding in your spice rack?

No! Dried herbs and spices are gluten-free. They very often have an anticaking agent added to them, but this is usually silicone-dioxide, calcium silicate, or sodium aluminum silica—all of which are gluten-free. Cheaper spices and imitation spices may have ground buckwheat or rice as filler, but seldom use wheat.

Seasoning packets, however, need to be checked carefully. Seasoning packets, like premixed taco seasoning, contain a mixture of spices and herbs, along with other carrier agents like sugar, salt, whey powder, starches, and flour. If the starches and flours originate from wheat, rye, barley, or oats, the product will not be gluten-free. Many sauce and seasoning packets that require thickening will use wheat flour as the thickening agent. All spice packets should be read carefully to determine whether or not they are safe to consume for those eating a gluten-free diet.

ESSENTIAL

Check online for spice mix recipes. Any commercial seasoning mix, whether a celebrity chef's signature seasoning, or a favorite Mexican restaurant's special blend, will likely have a close clone or copy available for you to try at home. There is no need to pay a higher price for a seasoning packet, especially if it may contain gluten.

To remove all uncertainty about the safety of seasoning packets, try mixing your own spices and herbs to create custom blends. Not only will this ensure that your ingredients are gluten-free, you can control the amount of spice and tailor the mix to your personal preference. If you want less salt or more spice, you have complete control. It is also cheaper to have a well-stocked spice rack than to purchase the individual seasoning blend packets. The chili powder in your spice rack can be used for making your award winning Chili Con Carne or some hot and spicy taco seasoning. This versatility is more economical than having a special packet on hand for each type of food you make.

Sharing a Kitchen with Gluten

Believe it or not, it is possible to share your kitchen with gluten, and not get sick. You do have to be very careful—and mindful—of what you are doing. But it is possible.

Begin with the basics: Keep products separated. If possible, store the products containing gluten and the gluten-free pantry items in different cupboards. If you don't have that much space, store the gluten-free items on a higher shelf and the products containing gluten on a lower shelf. If you keep the foods that contain gluten on the top shelf and crumbs fall while you are removing something from a package, the crumbs may contaminate the gluten-free foods. By storing the gluten-free items on top, you will eliminate the possibility of gluten cross-contamination.

Keep or buy condiments like mayonnaise, mustard, ketchup, and relish in squeeze bottles. Noncontact squeeze bottles are the best way to reduce cross-contamination when condiments are used for both gluten-free and gluten-filled foods. Just be extra cautious not to wipe the squeeze bottles against the bread. If the nozzle touches bread that contains gluten, it could make the condiment unsafe for those on a gluten-free diet. Don't be afraid to instruct your guests or family members on this point either, as it may not occur to them that there is a risk for cross-contamination if they do so.

For items that need to be scraped out of a container with a knife, like jam, peanut butter, and margarine, it is best to have clearly labeled, separate containers. Mark one "gluten-free" and one "regular" or use some other form of identification. When a knife is used to spread jam on a piece of wheat-based bread, and then it is used to remove more jam from the jar, the jam has become contaminated with gluten. Even that miniscule amount of gluten can be enough to make a person sick. By having dedicated gluten-free containers, you can control and eliminate cross-contamination. Be sure to label both the container and the lid so that you can still tell the difference between the regular and gluten-free even with the lid removed.

As discussed earlier in this chapter, some equipment is difficult to keep clean enough to share with gluten-containing foods, so it's better to use separate versions of some tools:

- Toasters
- Strainers and colanders
- Cutting boards
- Plastic mixing bowls

Be sure to keep any special gluten-free kitchen equipment separate from the equipment that regularly handles gluten-containing food. Storing them separately will eliminate confusion and prevent you from using the wrong one. When it comes to your health, it is always best to err on the side of caution.

CHAPTER 7

Buying Gluten-Free

It can be a little overwhelming to read labels at first, but as you get used to it, you will find that you are able to buy gluten-free foods nearly everywhere. And when it comes to baking, where the big decision used to be all-purpose flour or whole-wheat flour, you are now faced with buying multiple flours and starches to recreate your favorite recipes. This chapter will help you to make those purchases without breaking the bank. Gluten-free foods and baking supplies may be easier to find than you think.

At the Grocery Store

The place where you do the majority of your shopping right now, your local grocery store, is the place where you will still be purchasing most of your groceries, even on a gluten-free diet. When you walk into the grocery store, you are usually greeted with the produce department. That department is almost entirely gluten-free. Certain nonproduce items may be placed throughout this department, things like baked goods using seasonal fruit, but they will be easy to spot and avoid. All unprocessed fruits and vegetables are naturally gluten-free and should make up a large part of your diet. By increasing the number of unprocessed fruits and vegetables that you eat, either for on-the-go snacks or by consuming more meatless dishes and salads, you can still have a very flavorful and colorful diet.

ALERT

According to the USDA, half of your plate should contain fruits and vegetables. This requirement can be easily met on a gluten-free diet by loading up on unprocessed fruits and vegetables—foods that are naturally gluten-free.

When walking by the bakery department in a grocery store, just keep on walking. The smell of the bakery can be hard to resist, but rarely will the bakery contain anything that is safe for people on a gluten-free diet. If a grocery store does carry gluten-free baked items, the smaller market-share and longer turnaround times from oven to store usually require that they be stored in a freezer, so look for them there. Many stores also have a dedicated "natural foods" section, complete with freezers, so if you have no luck finding gluten-free items in the other aisles, try that area.

Now move on to the frozen foods section, whether it's in the conventional side of the store or a dedicated natural foods section. Again, if your grocery store carries gluten-free baked goods, keep an eye open while in the frozen foods section. The frozen foods section also holds a lot of naturally gluten-free items as well. Unprocessed seafood and meat—unbreaded, of course—can be gluten-free. Carefully read the ingredients to make sure, since they may have been marinated or injected with a solution that contains gluten. You can also find a lot of frozen vegetables, fruit, and of course, ice cream treats. Be sure to read the labels on ice cream. Some brands contain wheat-based filler and the ones that contain candy, cookie add-ins, or are already on a cone are off limits. You will have to do a lot more label reading while in the frozen foods section, so dress warmly. (You may be frustrated and bored with all this label reading, but keep it up! Soon it will be second nature to you.)

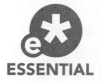

Less label reading will be required in the dairy aisle. All varieties of milk, margarine, and butter are gluten-free. That should make shopping in this aisle quite a bit easier. When it comes to cheese, most of the types of cheese that you find will be gluten-free. You will need to read the labels on preshredded cheese though, as some brands may use wheat-based anticaking agent to keep the shreds from sticking together. Cream cheese, sour cream, yogurt, and cottage cheese are all usually safe. Although the labels often read "modified food starch," this starch is most often derived from corn. When gluten-free labeling laws improve, the labels should begin identifying what type of grain the food starch is derived from, making it easier to identify hidden gluten in processed foods.

Generally speaking, it is more difficult to find gluten-free foods in the center aisles of a grocery store. Most of the items located there are processed and will require careful label reading. Some items, like rice, sugar, and canned beans, are gluten-free. Many other items, like seasoned rice packets, crackers, canned soup, and snack bars, are likely to contain gluten. Reading the fine print on labels can be a long process at first. Once you find a few items and brands that you know are gluten-free, double-checking the label will go much faster.

In larger grocery stores, however, you'll find a department that can be very helpful for those baking gluten-free—ethnic foods. In the ethnic foods department, or in ethnic food stores, you can very often find specialty flours that are used in gluten-free baking, and they are usually priced lower than in specialty stores:

- Rice flour, sweet rice flour (glutinous rice flour), and tapioca starch (also called tapioca flour) can all be purchased in the Asian food aisle or at an Asian market.
- Sorghum flour (also called jowar flour) and amaranth flour (also called rajagro flour) can be purchased in authentic Indian food stores.
- Mexican cuisine uses a lot of corn flour and cornmeal, so those flours can be found in that department.

Purchasing your flours in the authentic food aisles or in authentic markets can save a lot of money; however, be aware of increased cross-contamination possibilities.

In addition to carrying many naturally gluten-free products, many supermarkets now have a gluten-free section where they sell gluten-free pasta, cereal, and baking mixes. Some stores may even have a gluten-free frozen foods area, where you can buy frozen gluten-free bread, pizza crust, and bagels. Since the number of people that need to eat a gluten-free diet has increased over the last few years, the number of commercially available products has increased as well. This means that larger companies are starting to produce and sell gluten-free foods, and those foods are more readily available. If the neighborhood supermarket doesn't carry any gluten-free breads or cereals, talk to the manager to see if it is possible for them to stock some gluten-free items. When you are able to purchase gluten-free breads and cereals in the supermarket, the prices are generally lower than in health food stores. This is probably due to the large buying power of many large chain-owned supermarkets over independent health food stores.

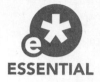

At Health Food Stores

Local health food stores are still incredibly helpful on a gluten-free journey. They will probably be the next place you shop after deciding to eat a gluten-free diet. Although many mainstream stores are finally beginning to carry gluten-free foods, health food stores have long carried many of the new-to-you gluten-free flours. Years ago, many people were not educated about the gluten-free diet, and really had no idea what the gluten-free diet entailed. Health food stores were the only places that carried all these different flours and gluten-free foods for a person diagnosed with celiac disease. Today, the number of gluten-free products available has jumped drastically. Instead of being able to only purchase rice flour at the health food store, you are able to buy sorghum and quinoa flours as well. Add to that all the gluten-free baking mixes and frozen breads, muffins, and pizza crusts that are now available, the health food store is a great resource.

Whether you are looking for a variety of gluten-free flours, xanthan gum, cereals, baking mixes, or crackers, you will be able to find them at the health food store. One upside to health food stores is that the staff is usually knowledgeable on the gluten-free products that they stock and is able to help you discern what is safe for you to eat. The downside to purchasing your gluten-free products from a health food store, however, is that the prices are normally higher than elsewhere.

Bakeries

Generally speaking, your neighborhood bakery is off limits when you are on a gluten-free diet, because they do all of their baking using wheat flour. There may be a few bakeries, however, that offer some gluten-free baked goods. You need to talk to the manager at the bakery and find out what procedures they use to ensure that the gluten-free goods are not cross-contaminated from the wheat-based products. If they are mixed and baked on the same equipment, it is not a good idea to indulge in those baked goods. A bakery that has wheat flour flying around everywhere would be very difficult to clean well enough to not cross-contaminate the gluten-free baked goods.

Fortunately, some bakeries have dedicated gluten-free facilities and equipment. As long as the bakery only bakes with gluten-free flours, the cakes and cookies they produce should be the perfect delectable delight to treat yourself or a loved one. You can find a list of gluten-free bakeries online at *www.celiacrestaurantguide.com*.

Shopping Online

Online purchasing has become a mainstream shopping method for many people. Whether you are looking for that impossible-to-find gift for a child, a customized wall hanging, car parts, or gluten-free food, all of them can be found with a few clicks of the mouse. Retail locations are limited by the store inventory, and no store stocks every brand of every gluten-free product available. But the Internet does. By shopping online and perusing the various retailers without leaving your desk chair, you will be able to find almost every brand and almost every product available. The variety of items available includes pasta, cereal, cosmetics, baking mixes, as well as some of those hard-to-find gluten-free flours.

FACT

Many websites have a great selection of gluten-free items available. Here are a few: *www.celiac.com/glutenfreemall/, www.glutenfree .com, www.kinnikinnick.com, www.bobsredmill.com/flours-meals/,* and *www.amazon.com*.

Due to your geographic location, you may have a hard time finding gluten-free flours and prepared food at your local stores. Cities and towns with higher populations will usually have a better selection than small-town stores. If you have a hard time finding gluten-free flours where you live, ordering online is definitely an option. Many gluten-free manufacturers have websites that list where their items can be purchased, or you may be able to purchase directly from their online shop.

Buying in Bulk

Often items purchased online can be bought in larger quantities. This is especially helpful once you find something that works well for your family. On Amazon.com, for example, when you order a case of pasta, cereal, or cookies, you get a price break over the regular price. Gluten-free foods are expensive, so before making any purchases in bulk, be sure that whatever you are buying is something that you or your family will actually use. Even a good online deal, one that saves money, is a waste of money if no one wants to eat it. If only one person in your family is on a gluten-free diet, or you are single, you can still order in bulk without the extra going to waste as long as the food keeps long enough. So many people are eating gluten-free for different reasons that, chances are, you know someone else that eats a diet without gluten as well. Whether it is a family member, friend, coworker, neighbor, or fellow member of a gluten-free support group, you can probably find someone interested in saving money by splitting a large bulk order with you.

When ordering gluten-free food in bulk, there are a few things to keep in mind.

1. **Flour is heavy.** The price tag on a 60-pound bag of flour may sound great, but you have to factor in the shipping costs before determining if it is a good deal for you.
2. **Foods have expiration dates.** All food, including gluten-free food, has a "best before" date. You cannot purchase a whole case of cookies thinking that you will now be set for the next ten years. No matter how the cookies are packaged or stored, they will eventually go bad and become

unsafe to eat. You need to order only what can reasonably be consumed in the next few weeks or months.

3. **You need to store it somewhere.** Make sure that you have room for all the bulk items that you are ordering. Flours are best stored in the fridge or freezer or they can become rancid. If you do not have an extra fridge or freezer to store 200 pounds of flour in, do not purchase 200 pounds of flour. Only order what you have room to store properly. If you leave all your flours on the shelves, and they become rancid, ordering them in bulk will not have saved you any money.

4. **Look local.** Unless you live down the street from a gluten-free food manufacturer, you may think there is nowhere you can buy in bulk locally. However, a lot of places in your neighborhood may be accommodating if you ask. There are places that purchase flours in bulk, and repackage them to sell them to the customer. There are also places where you can purchase flours and baking mixes by the scoop. Both of these places already have accounts with the manufacturer and order their products in large quantities. If you ask, you may be able to purchase large quantities from them, at a discounted price, before they repackage it to sell. This would allow you to purchase in bulk and save on the shipping cost.

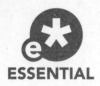

ESSENTIAL

Major brand-name products, the kind that you grew up eating and have traditionally been made with wheat flour, have begun to appear on the gluten-free shelves in the grocery stores. In recent years, gluten-free versions of Bisquick, Betty Crocker cake mixes, and Rice Krispies have been brought to market. These products are quickly becoming new favorites among the gluten-free community.

Farmers' Markets and Outdoor Sellers

Your local farmers' market may be more accommodating to those living a gluten-free lifestyle than you might expect. All of the fresh fruits and vegetables will be gluten-free, and many may even be organic. The producers that sell at these outdoor markets take great pride in bringing their customers products that are superior to what they will find in their grocery store.

They are very knowledgeable about their ingredients and what goes into the final product. Farmers selling processed foods like meats, jellies, and sauces will know the ingredient list for their goods, and they will also have a complete understanding of the manufacturing process. They will know if their food has come into contact with gluten and they will be able to warn you away from dangerous items. Talk to the sellers. Ask them about their product, and the processes they use. Not only will this enhance your farmers' market shopping experience, it will allow you to make educated decisions about whether or not the food is safe for you to eat.

ALERT

If a vendor can't answer your questions, has a disorganized setup, or seems unknowledgeable about his or her own products, don't make any purchases there!

You may also find vendors selling gluten-free baked goods at an outdoor market. In these venues, be sure to ask plenty of questions of anyone selling products labeled gluten-free. Keep in mind that the labeling guidelines that large manufacturers must comply with do not all apply to small-market retailers. Don't forget to ask them questions about their manufacturing process. Is the kitchen they bake in used exclusively for gluten-free foods, or are there also wheat-based flours and products in the kitchen? If so, be sure to ask them what steps they take to prevent cross-contamination and what they do to ensure that their gluten-free products are indeed free of all gluten. After talking with the seller, use your best judgment. Ask yourself if you feel confident that their products are, indeed, completely free of all gluten. Remember, even trace amounts of gluten can trigger a number of unpleasant symptoms. A good vendor will be able to answer your questions to your satisfaction.

CHAPTER 8

Gluten-Free on the Road

When planning your next vacation or business trip, whether you are traveling by train, plane, or car, don't let the fact that you are on a gluten-free diet deter you from going and having a great time. With a little bit of planning, you can still have a fantastic time while maintaining a gluten-free diet. The key to any successful trip will be in good planning, so start organizing your meals long before leaving the house.

Tips on Eating Gluten-Free While Traveling

Regardless of your mode of travel, or your destination, begin your trip by packing some gluten-free snacks to take along. Naturally gluten-free food, like fruit and nuts, which are easy to pick up at any store, are a great snack to pack wherever you are headed. Snacks that are labeled "gluten-free" like Larabars, Sesame Snaps, or gluten-free pretzels are also great to take along since they do not require any special care when packing them. Just throw these items into a suitable bag and you are ready to go. Gluten-free muffins are another good snack to take along. They can also serve double-duty as your breakfast while you are away from home. Muffins can be baked with dried fruits, nuts, and whole grains, loading them with nutrition for a great-tasty breakfast or snack. Muffins don't need to be kept in the refrigerator so they are a good option when looking for a healthy snack to take on your trip, but they may need a little more protection. Storing them in small, rigid, plastic containers will help keep them from getting squished in your travel bag.

Traveling by plane? Be sure to request a gluten-free meal when booking your tickets. Most carriers should be able to fulfill your request, or if not, they will let you know. Also be sure to notify them or remind them of your request at least a few days before your departure. Although the airline may offer a gluten-free meal, it is still recommended that you pack your own snacks. Remember, be prepared, just in case the airline has an error or communication breakdown and does not have a gluten-free meal ready for you. As long as snacks are wrapped in a resealable plastic bag and compliant with TSA regulations, they should be safe to take on an airplane. You don't want to find yourself 30,000 feet above the earth, on an eight-hour flight, with only the airline's complimentary crackers to tide you over—they won't be gluten-free. As long as you always carry some gluten-free snacks with you, you will never be stuck in that situation.

If you are traveling by train, it is best to pack your meals before departing. Amtrak, for example, does not supply meals that are specifically designated as "gluten-free." The meals they offer may not actually contain any gluten, but they may have become contaminated from the preparation process, preventing them from being labeled "gluten-free." In Canada, Via Rail does offer gluten-free meals, but only on certain routes and only if they are given ten days' notice. Like Amtrak, you are welcome to bring along your own gluten-free foods.

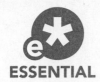

If you're packing up the car and hitting the open road, embarking on your own road trip, invest in an electric cooler, one that can plug into your vehicle's 12-volt cigarette lighter or auxiliary power outlet. As long as your vehicle is running, the cooler will keep gluten-free sandwiches, salads, cut-up raw vegetables, cheese, and drinks cool and you won't need to worry about them spoiling along the way. An adapter can also be purchased to use with these coolers so that they can be plugged into a regular household outlet once you stop for the day or get to your final destination. Don't leave them plugged into the vehicle's battery when the engine is not running as this can discharge the battery, turning your road trip into a "stay-cation."

Other great snacks to pack for the hours spent on the road include fruit, gluten-free muffins, cookies, or crackers, candy, chips, gluten-free granola bars or pretzels, and nuts. Packing your own food will ensure that you are eating gluten-free and it will lower the food expenses for your trip, freeing up funds for some serious vacationing.

Locating Gluten-Free-Friendly Restaurants

Before heading out, whether for the day or the week, it is best to do some research. Finding out whether the area you will be traveling to has a local celiac or gluten-intolerant support group is a great starting point. Many local gluten-intolerant support groups list the restaurants in their area that offer gluten-free menu options or are at least willing to accommodate those eating a gluten-free diet. By searching online, you can very often find reviews of the local restaurants. You can then decide for yourself if you feel that the restaurant can serve your needs properly and safely. You can search for a local Gluten Intolerance Group of North America (GIG) at *www.gluten.net*.

Many restaurants have websites that promote their menu online. Often, if the restaurant has a gluten-free menu, they will post that information on their website as well. If they do not have a dedicated gluten-free menu, they may have a section for allergy information or instruct their customers to discuss their concerns with the serving staff or request to speak to a manager. Don't be shy; restaurants are in the service industry and all the staff should be happy to address your concerns.

If you have a particular restaurant in mind, but are unable to find any information online regarding their menu, be sure to phone the restaurant ahead of time and talk to the manager to see if they are able to meet your dietary requirements. It is always best to visit restaurants during their slow times. This may mean stopping for an early lunch or supper. Serving and kitchen staff will not be as busy during these times, and will be able to give your order their full, considerate attention.

Beware Cross-Contamination

Many restaurants that feature an allergy-information sheet cannot guarantee that their food is gluten-free. It's difficult for them to prevent gluten-contamination while the dish is being prepared in a busy commercial kitchen. What the allergy-information sheet says is that the food, as prepared, does not contain any gluten. The chance of cross-contamination is still a reality so you have to decide whether or not the risk of cross-contamination is a risk you want to take. Again, talk to the serving staff or ask to see the manager to have your concerns addressed. Reputable establishments will understand the special preparations necessary and be able to explain the steps they take in the kitchen to prevent contamination.

Websites and Apps

Whether you travel within the United States or are journeying overseas, the Celiac Restaurant Guide (*www.celiacrestaurantguide.com*) has the answers for you. You can search by state and city within the United States, or you can search by country and city for foreign travel. You can search for restaurants that offer both gluten-free and wheat-based food on their menu, or a restaurant or bakery that offers 100 percent gluten-free items.

Already connected to the information age with a smartphone, portable handheld device, or tablet computer? Check for and download applications (apps) that can provide you with a list of celiac-friendly restaurants based on your current geographic location. There are many apps available to help you with your gluten-free dining experience. Bookmark or download any that you find helpful. Gluten Free Registry (*www.glutenfreeregistry.com*) is a free app that will assist you in finding restaurants, grocers, and bakeries that offer gluten-free food in a quick, efficient manner. By simply clicking on the state or province and city where you are, it compiles a list of nearby restaurants and bakeries that offer gluten-free menus.

Find Me Gluten Free (*www.findmeglutenfree.com*) is another fantastic free app that locates gluten-free restaurants, bakeries, grocery stores, and cafés. Whether you are looking for fast food, a place to relax with a light meal, or a fine dining experience, this app will find the place for you. When you type in your desired location, it will show you the restaurants in the area that fit your criteria as well as automatically providing directions to get there. Businesses are tagged with the special gluten-free features that they offer, such as pizza, pasta, bread, or a dedicated gluten-free facility. With tools like these at your fingertips, finding a place to sit, relax, and have a satisfying gluten-free meal while traveling is easy and convenient.

Ordering at Restaurants

If you can't choose a gluten-free-friendly restaurant, you can still manage your experience in a safe way. After all, sometimes you won't get to choose the restaurant. Friends, family, or business associates may make the decision on where you will be dining, leaving you without the option of having a gluten-free menu available. Don't let this stress you. There are still plenty of options available on the regular menu. You will just need to use all the research and self-education you've done to make safe food choices and minimize your risk.

You may have to avoid appetizers altogether, as many of them are breaded and fried. For a starter, stick with green salads with olive oil or balsamic vinegar dressings on the side. Be sure that your salad does not have, and has not been tossed with, croutons. If a salad has croutons sprinkled on top, or has them throughout the salad, the salad has now been contaminated with gluten. If the salad you order comes with croutons on it, explain to your server that, for health reasons, you need to have a salad without any bread products on it and ask them for a replacement.

ALERT

If you order a salad and it arrives with croutons in it, have the server bring you a new salad before removing the gluten-contaminated salad from your table. This will ensure the kitchen is sending you a new salad, and not just removing the croutons before re-serving you the same salad. Explain politely what you are doing if the server asks or tries to remove the salad.

For main dishes, avoid any foods that are deep-fried. Even if they are not breaded, they may be contaminated with gluten by sharing the deep fryer with foods that are battered. Look for beef, chicken, pork, or seafood that is roasted, grilled, broiled, or baked. Always be very clear with your server, making sure that they understand that for medical reasons, you need to have a meal that is free from gluten. Foods like roast chicken and grilled steak are great alternatives when going out to eat. Be sure to ask your server if the meats have been marinated or rubbed with a seasoning, and to be sure that those seasonings are also gluten-free. Baked potatoes and roasted vegetables are wonderful, healthy side dishes that are also, generally, gluten-free.

Processed and breaded foods have a higher chance of containing gluten, since gluten is often used as a filler and a binder during their production. So stay away from chicken fingers, breaded shrimp, and mozzarella sticks. French fries are sometimes coated in seasoned flour coating, so it is best to ask your server if their French fries are gluten-free. Also ask if they are fried in a dedicated fryer, not the same one that fries breaded chicken fingers, for example.

Although those triple-layer chocolate cakes and cheesecake desserts look extremely temping, you will most likely need to avoid those when eating in a restaurant. However, you do not need to say no to dessert all together. If you communicate your need for a gluten-free dessert with your server, you can usually get a fruit salad or a scoop of ice cream to end your meal.

Being able to order a gluten-free meal from a regular menu doesn't need to be stressful. It can be a very nice dining experience. Again, communication with your server, and sometimes the manager, will ensure that the kitchen staff knows and understands your dietary needs. If you feel apprehensive about ordering at a restaurant, Triumph Dining (*www.triumphdining.com*) has laminated dining cards that can be purchased online. When you go out to eat, you simply show your server your dining card, and it clearly states what you can and cannot eat. This is an easy way to communicate your special dietary needs with the server and the kitchen staff, and helps them understand how they can safely serve you.

The number of people that are realizing that they need to eat a gluten-free diet is on the rise. Restaurants are responding by educating their staff about gluten, and how to safely prepare foods for those who cannot eat it. You may feel awkward or rude by peppering your server with questions, but if your health or the health of someone you love is at stake, try to keep that in mind. As long as you are inquiring politely and reasonably, there is no reason the server or manager should be annoyed. Some restaurants put in an amazing effort to serve their customers who are on a gluten-free diet by ordering in freshly baked gluten-free breads and desserts. Doing this allows gluten-free meals to be almost indistinguishable from their standard menu fare.

Quick and Healthy Snacks on the Go

Sometimes, you just don't have the time or the energy to prepare food to take along before heading out on a journey. That's understandable, as life is busy and there is a lot to do even on the slow days. In those cases, a quick trip to the grocery store, or even a gas station, can help you find suitable snacks to tame your hunger until the next meal.

It might not be the healthiest choice, but at a gas station you can usually find candy, nuts, chips, and drinks that do not contain any gluten. These are not the ideal snacks and it's not a good idea to rely on them on a regular basis, but they will get you out of a bind.

To find healthier alternatives, stop at a grocery store. While out on the road, instead of looking for the usual fast-food places when your tummy starts to rumble, look for the stores where the locals shop. You can usually find gluten-free crackers, cheese, yogurt, ready-to-eat fruit and vegetables, as well as prepared salads that do not contain gluten. If you are traveling by vehicle and have an electric cooler with you, you can also use this opportunity to stock up the cooler with healthy gluten-free foods that you can eat after you've been on the road for a few more hours.

Staying at a Hotel or Out of Town with Friends

Common considerations when booking a hotel room include things like location, price, nearby attractions, and, if you have kids, a great pool or water park. When you are on a gluten-free diet, look for a few other things that will make your stay a little easier, and cheaper, as well.

Check if the hotel you are booking has in-room refrigerators. Having a refrigerator in your room will allow you to store yogurt, milk, salads, fruits, and vegetables close by. Many simple meals can be prepared with these fresh ingredients, reducing or eliminating the need for finding a restaurant with gluten-free menu items for every meal. This can save both time and money. If you are unable to find a hotel that offers a refrigerator in the room, bring along a portable electric cooler. They aren't as big and can't store as much food, but they are very convenient and will keep your food fresh. Just be sure that you have an adapter for plugging into a standard wall outlet.

Other room amenities like a microwave oven or coffee maker also make it easier to prepare meals from purchased ingredients. If the room does not have a microwave, check the pool area, the breakfast area, or other common areas to see if one is available. Use the microwave to make a plate of gluten-free nachos or to heat up a gluten-free frozen dinner.

Book a hotel that serves a free continental breakfast, and you are well on your way to having your gluten-free breakfast taken care of. Continental breakfasts traditionally consist of gluten-containing items like muffins, bagels, and toast, but most hotels that offer them will also feature some naturally gluten-free items like yogurt, fresh fruit, and coffee or juice. If your hotel offers a free continental breakfast, make a quick stop at a local grocery store that carries gluten-free breads and cereals before checking in. Armed with your own gluten-free bread, bagels, muffins, or cereal, together with the naturally gluten-free fare offered by the hotel, you will have a fantastic breakfast that will keep you full for hours. The little butters, jams, and spreads that the hotel offers in their breakfast area are nice, individual sized portions that won't be contaminated from the breads and baked goods that the hotel offers. Avoid the hotel's waffle maker, and it is probably best to avoid the toaster as well. That is, unless you purchase toaster bags (*www.amazon.com/dp/ B0012XGM92*), which are heatproof reusable bags that you slide your bread into before placing it in the toaster. However, commercially available gluten-free bread loaves and bagels have improved dramatically in quality and flavor and no longer require toasting to make them edible.

If you buy a gluten-free cereal, use one of the bowls from the hotel's breakfast area and use the milk that they have by their other beverages. Use your imagination and you can have a quick, simple, nutritious, and filling gluten-free breakfast.

Camping Gluten-Free

Camping is a great, affordable way to travel. You get to enjoy lakes, rivers, forests, and parks and the thrill of living as close to the wilderness as a modern pioneer can get. Every campground has a unique character defined by the natural features and local culture that surrounds it. It might seem difficult to stay gluten-free in this type of setting, but again, with the proper planning, you won't have any problems. You may find that it's even easier staying gluten-free while camping than it is during other forms of travel.

Planning and preparation are important first steps. Obviously the plan will change depending on the type of camping. Hiking the Appalachian Trail or some other pack-out-what-you-pack-in back-country trail will require different planning from setting out in a thirty-five-foot recreational vehicle with a kitchenette, stove, microwave, and refrigerator.

Experience will be the best guide here. If you are a veteran of either type of camping, you will already have a good idea how you will manage to remain gluten-free. In the case of RV travel, you can purge the gluten out of your mobile home and restock it, paring down your goods to fit inside the smaller refrigerator and the reduced storage spaces. In this sense, RVing is a lot like staying in hotels. Keeping your RV gluten-free should follow the same basic rules used in a home kitchen. If you are going to allow regular bread, or other gluten-containing foods, into your camper, keep them separated, keep them on lower shelves, and make sure you have separate containers for spreads like preserves and jellies or peanut butter. Stock your RV like you would your house, taking the smaller spaces into consideration.

Smaller campers that tow behind a vehicle can use the same principles. Things get more difficult when you start getting into folding tent-trailers and tents. For this type of camping, an electric cooler is going to be essential. Large plastic bins can be used to store other food and ingredients. It will be more difficult to keep gluten-containing items separate in these close quarters to prevent cross contamination, so it might be a good idea to eliminate gluten entirely. Pack the type of food you like to eat.

Gluten-free chips, crackers, snack bars, sausages, or other processed meats can all safely be transported and stored in campers and camping bins. Prepare some salads ahead of time and store them in large resealable plastic bags that can be thrown away once they are empty. You can pack raw meats, but take care to prevent foodborne illnesses from getting hold before you have a chance to cook your meal. Store them at proper temperatures.

Backpacking will be the greatest challenge. Packing bread may be a very poor option. Gluten-containing bread will need to coexist in a small pack that is constantly in motion, getting squished against other pack items, possibly leading to the bag tearing. Gluten-free loaves are typically smaller than regular bread and packing several to make up the equivalent amount may add undue weight to your pack. Again, experience will be the best guide. Keep an open mind and be willing to experiment. You will find a solution that works for whatever type of camping you choose to pursue.

CHAPTER 9

Party Time!

Any kind of restricted diet makes eating at restaurants, or at friends' houses, more difficult. When you are on a gluten-free diet, meeting up with friends at a restaurant at the last minute is a challenge. Visiting friends and family can be just as difficult since many people do not fully understand all the places where gluten can be found. Fewer understand the effects gluten can have on a person who is on a gluten-free diet. Fear not, your social life is not over. It is possible to socialize with friends and family while maintaining a gluten-free diet.

Letting Hosts Know (Nicely!)

Social gatherings of any kind usually revolve around food. Heading to a friend's house for a weekend barbecue, going to a niece's birthday party, or attending an old friend's wedding will all contain a full meal at which the host will expect the guests to enjoy the food that has been prepared. It is generally considered impolite or rude to refuse food at these times since one of the hallmarks of good hospitality is ensuring guests are well fed before leaving. This can place people on a gluten-free diet in a difficult position. Without being sure the food served will be safe for you to eat, you are faced with two equally unpleasant options: Refuse to attend or refuse to eat.

Even though the last thing you want to do is draw attention to your dietary needs, the best way to handle this situation is to inform the host ahead of time of your dietary restrictions. If you do not discuss your diet with the host ahead of time, you put the host in an awkward position when you arrive and are unable to eat anything that has been prepared for you.

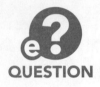

QUESTION

How do you "break the ice" about your diet?
You can respond to invitations by asking if there is anything that you can bring, and offer to bring a gluten-free version or variant of whatever is needed. Politely explain that you have to eat a gluten-free diet, and that you may get ill if you eat any foods containing even small amounts of gluten. Also use this conversation to educate the host on common sources of gluten and cross-contamination.

Admittedly, it can be awkward talking about dietary restrictions with someone who is kind enough to host you, but it is best for everyone if you notify the host ahead of time that you cannot eat anything that contains wheat, rye, barley, or oats. Use this opportunity to educate the host about the gluten-free diet; where gluten is found, and, more importantly, the unexpected places it hides. Do not expect your host to know about hidden gluten sources or cross-contamination. Be patient with them and remember that this was all new for you once, too. Take the time to share the lessons you learned when you began a gluten-free diet and the things you discovered through your research. Again, if your host seems confused or concerned, offer to bring your own food or a favorite gluten-free dish to share with the group.

ALERT

Croutons, imitation bacon bits, and salad dressings may contain gluten. A great way to serve a garden salad is by having small bowls with those items on the side and people can add toppings to their own salads. This will prevent cross-contamination with gluten and make the first course safe for everyone to enjoy.

If you are attending a formal occasion like a graduation or wedding, and the hosts are unable to answer your questions regarding the meal, ask for the name of the caterer and, at least a week before the event, contact the caterer directly. There may be an additional cost to prepare a special plate for you, which you should be willing to compensate the host for. Ask them which, if any, menu items that will be served are gluten-free. This will give you a very good indication of whether there will be enough gluten-free items to make a complete meal. If the caterer responds by saying very few items are gluten-free, feel free to eat before the event or bring along some of your own food. It is best to keep a small portable snack with you any time you attend a formal event, just in case plans change and there are no safe alternatives for you to eat. In large, catered, formal settings you may encounter a dish, like a cheese platter, that is gluten-free but by the way it is served, surrounded by crackers, makes it unsafe for you to eat. In these cases, having a snack on hand will save the day.

Being a Good and Gracious Gluten-Free Guest

When you are invited to any function that involves food, it is important to be polite and considerate when letting others know about your restricted diet. Do not expect them to change an entire menu just for you. Openly communicate with them, and realize that you may need to eat before attending, or bring your own food along to ensure that you have something safe to eat.

Before attending any event, ask the host what foods they plan to serve. If you are unsure about any dishes, ask for the recipe or ingredient list. This will help you determine whether or not the food may contain gluten. For example, if the meat marinade contains soy or Worcestershire sauce, the item may contain gluten since not all brands of soy sauce or Worcestershire sauce are gluten-free. If a salad contains crunchy fried onions, the dish will not be gluten-free, since those onions are battered in a wheat-based batter before deep-frying.

By asking for the menu ahead of time, your intention should not be to try to deter the host from preparing what they intended. Rather, use the information to prepare yourself by knowing what will be safe for you to eat and what will not be safe. If you know the menu ahead of time, and know what food will be safe for you to eat, you can prevent an uncomfortable moment while the food is being served. It also gives the host a chance to rethink their menu or possibly add more naturally gluten-free items, or to make small changes to their existing menu to make the current items gluten-free. Do not expect a host to make a fully gluten-free meal for you; rather, educate yourself about what you can eat, and just stick to that. Never make you host feel guilty for not providing you with a gluten-free meal, at least not if you ever want to be invited back.

While talking to the host about what the gluten-free diet all entails, be sure to emphasise the simple things. Let the host know that unprocessed foods, like fresh fruits and vegetables, are naturally gluten-free. One does not have to hunt down foods specifically labeled "gluten-free" in order to serve a person on a gluten-free diet, so offer up some suggestions. A fruit platter served with a yogurt-based dip is naturally gluten-free, as is a vegetable platter served with hummus, and platters like these can be enjoyed by everyone attending. A baked potato buffet, where everyone loads their own baked potatoes with a variety of supplied toppings, is perfect for everyone, including those eating gluten-free. Unprocessed meats, like beefsteak, salmon fillets, pork loin, and chicken breast are all gluten-free, as long as they are prepared properly.

If attending a barbecue or gathering, offer to bring a dish for everyone to enjoy that is also gluten-free. Bring along a large salad or dessert to share with everyone, and then you will know that you have at least one safe, gluten-free dish or dessert that you can eat.

Navigating Around the Potluck Table

One of the most difficult meals to navigate is a potluck. With guests expected to bring their own dish to the event, there is no control over the contents of the food served. There is usually very little information on the ingredients used, and less on how the food has been prepared. If you know the group of people that is hosting the potluck, suggest they ask everyone to write out the recipe, with ingredients, for each dish they bring. Ask them to write the recipe on an index card and display that card alongside the dish on the table. With the prevalence of food intolerances these days, others at the potluck might also appreciate knowing what is in the food they are about to eat. Or, people might just like to copy the recipe to make it themselves! With an ingredient list next to each dish, it will be easier for you to decide if the dish is safe for you to eat.

ESSENTIAL

At a potluck, ask if you may fill up your plate first. It may feel odd to make this request but, at an informal buffet like a potluck, spoons and serving utensils are often exchanged between dishes. Food may accidentally drop into neighboring bowls, causing a gluten-free dish to become contaminated. By quietly and discretely serving yourself first, you ensure the gluten-free food on your plate is, indeed, still gluten-free.

If you have absolutely no control over the potluck, stick to the dishes with the least amount of processed food. Salads without dressings, roasted meats, and fruit or vegetable platters are all safe places to start. Be sure to bring along one or two dishes yourself, because then you will know that those are safe for you to eat. If you have close friends or family attending the potluck, ask them to bring a gluten-free dish as well. Only having two or three dishes that you know are safe for you to eat is better than guessing at the ingredients and taking a chance on getting sick.

You could also pack a picnic-style meal for yourself and take it along to the potluck, totally eliminating the worries of hidden ingredients and cross-contamination. No one will mind if you are eating something else as they will just be glad that you still came to enjoy the company. Potluck meals are difficult to navigate while on a gluten-free diet, but don't let that stop you from attending them. They are fun, social times at which you get to connect with family and friends. It would be a shame to restrict these relationships just because of a restricted, gluten-free diet.

What to Bring and Share

The easiest way to know what is safe to eat at any event that revolves around food is to prepare and bring a dish or two along. Anytime you are invited to a dinner or potluck, after accepting the invitation, immediately ask, "What can I bring?" Your offer to contribute to the meal will likely be met with gratitude and, by preparing a dish, you ensure at least one safe item will be available for you to eat. You will also be contributing to the meal with a dish that everyone can enjoy, not just those on a gluten-free diet.

Eating gluten-free can cost a lot more than eating a regular, wheat-based diet and you may think this extra expense will prevent you from bringing a dish or two to share with everyone. If cost is an issue, consider bringing simple dishes that use fresh fruits or vegetables. You can bring coleslaw, broccoli salad, taco salad, or a Jell-O salad. There is a large number of salads that are naturally gluten-free and do not contain any special gluten-free ingredients.

If you want to bring a meat dish, you can prepare baked chicken wings; a juicy, slow cooked roast; or even meatballs in sweet and sour sauce. By keeping the foods simple to prepare and transport, and being sure to use gluten-free ingredients, you can bring a dish that everyone will love. They won't even notice that you, or they, are eating gluten-free. Your friend may make amazing chicken wings but since many ingredients, like soy sauce or Worcestershire sauce, may not be gluten-free, the wings would not be safe to eat. But, if you make the same recipe, ensuring that the ingredients used are gluten-free, no one will be able to tell the difference, and the wings could be enjoyed by everyone. Small, simple substitutions can make a dish that was unsafe for you to eat into a gluten-free meal to enjoy.

ALERT

Always read the ingredient list on ice cream containers carefully. Some manufacturers add wheat flour to the ice cream to help prevent ice crystals from forming. Gluten containing cookie bits or candy bar chunks are often added to ice cream, contaminating it with gluten and making it unsafe for those with celiac disease or gluten intolerance.

Desserts, too, can be made naturally gluten-free without requiring any special store-bought gluten-free items. Fruit salad, flourless chocolate cake, flourless peanut butter cookies, or pavlova—a decadent meringue dessert—are all naturally gluten-free. Everyone will like these sweet, tasty, and simple-to-prepare desserts. For summertime get-togethers, have a quart of gluten-free ice cream and some sundae toppings on hand. This simple dessert takes no time to prepare and everyone, gluten-free or otherwise, can enjoy it.

By being willing to provide food and assist in its preparation, you can ensure that you will have great gluten-free meals at all your social gatherings.

Explaining Your Diet

Explaining your new gluten-free diet should not be difficult as long as you have supportive friends and family who are concerned about your health and are willing to listen. Most of them have already heard the term "gluten-free" by now, but they may not realize what adopting this diet entails or why it's necessary. There is a lot to learn about gluten-free living so don't expect them to remember everything the first time it is explained to them.

The first thing they need to understand is that eating gluten-free, for those with celiac disease or a gluten intolerance, is not a diet of choice, but rather, a diet of necessity. It is not a fad or a phase, or based on some trend started by a celebrity. It's more of a medical prescription to address the fact that your body cannot tolerate the proteins found in gluten. These proteins are simply making you ill, and to fix the problem you must avoid all contact with them. A gluten-free diet is the only way to eliminate the hazard they present to your health. It might be easiest for them to think of gluten in terms of something they are more familiar with. Drawing comparisons to severe nut or seafood allergies, lactose intolerance, or even the lethal responses some people have to bee stings, can help them understand that celiac disease, or gluten intolerance, exists next to a whole spectrum of food disorders and health problems that requires careful lifestyle consideration. Would this person tell someone with a seafood allergy to just get over it and eat the crabs' legs already? Probably not.

Once someone understands that gluten-free diets are restrictive by nature and are not a choice, they may begin to stress about how to feed you when it's time to throw a party. It's not abnormal for someone to exclaim with exasperation, "I have nothing for you to eat." Quickly assure them that they do have something you can eat, and begin a conversation focused on helping them understand several things. They will need to understand how prevalent gluten is in modern food products. Take some items off their pantry shelf and go through the list of ingredients pointing out the harmful ones. If possible, show them an example of a label that contains a warning like "May contain traces of tree nuts, soy, or wheat" so they become familiar with how to read food packaging and they can get a sense that you are not unique or alone in the world. While you will have to make it clear where gluten may be hiding, you can also assure them that they don't need to spend too much time worrying about it, since there are many gluten-free options available. However, be clear that anything made from wheat, rye, barley, and oats will produce ill effects, even if it is only used as a subingredient in a product. Let them know that even a small amount of gluten can make you sick. If you can get them to understand this one point, the conversation can be considered a success. Again, the point is not for the person to change his or her party menu for you, but for them to communicate clearly with you about what's being served and how it was prepared.

Asking your family and friends to respect your new lifestyle should not be difficult, if they can truly care about your health and well-being. They may still doubt the necessity of your new diet, they may even roll their eyes once or twice, but ask them to refrain from the belief that "a little won't hurt you" when, in fact, ingesting a tiny amount of gluten is as dangerous as ingesting a large amount. Gently remind them that they wouldn't think that way about someone with a peanut or seafood allergy. Also remind them that, while people with lactose intolerance can take a dietary supplement that enables them to eat dairy products, no such pill exists for gluten.

Citing statistics and explaining how common celiac disease and gluten-sensitivity are may help them understand the seriousness of your condition. It may also help them understand dietary choices—or other unexplained behavior—they have seen in their other friends. Along with statistics, explaining that there is a broad spectrum of other disorders that are helped by eating a gluten-free diet may actually trigger a change in their own diet, leading them to better health and wellness. If you are discussing celiac disease and gluten-free living with close relatives, you can inform them that the condition has a genetic component and that they may also be affected. According to medical experts, first-degree relatives, like mothers, fathers, brothers, and sisters, have a 1 in 22 chance of also having celiac disease. In second-degree relatives the numbers are slightly lower, but still significant. Cousins, uncles, aunts, nieces, and nephews have a 1 in 39 chance of also having celiac disease.

ESSENTIAL

No one will be as concerned about or take your health as seriously as you will. It may be surprising when close friends and family members respond disrespectfully upon first hearing about your need to eat gluten-free. This may be due to a sense of fear and insecurity and their lack of understanding. Try not to take it personally and try not to let their response damage your relationship.

No matter who you are explaining your diet to, whether it be friends, family, or hosts, be prepared to repeatedly answer a lot of similar questions. Take time to answer the questions politely and make sure that they feel free to repeat questions that they are not clear about. Asking and answering questions more than once is the best way to make sure the information gets locked away in a person's memory. If living gluten-free is not a priority for someone, they can't be expected to remember all the hints, tips, and ideas you've offered in the past.

Yes, party time will be more difficult when you try to keep gluten away. You can't avoid it but you can make it easier and more of a party for everyone. Planning, preparation, and open communication are simple steps you can take to make sure that the next get-together is fun, safe, and even a little educational for everyone.

CHAPTER 10

Gluten-Free Kids

It is a huge lifestyle change to begin a gluten-free diet for an adult. It can be difficult and frustrating to switch over to a life without gluten. For kids, the situations can be even more difficult. Their social life revolves around school, birthday parties, and playdates, and all of those activities will involve food, whether it's birthday cake or snack time. These are times when a child who has to eat gluten-free may feel left out or different. Yet, with a few hints and tips, these feelings can be minimized or prevented. Create a team to help you deal with your child's gluten-free diet, including teachers, parents, and friends, and together you can all make the transition to a gluten-free diet easier on your child.

How to Help Your Child Deal with the Changes

Making the change to a gluten-free diet is a huge undertaking for anyone, but it is especially difficult with children. Children may not understand why certain food makes them sick; they don't have the same level of understanding that an adult does. They may not see the connection between that delicious soft pretzel at the mall and the tummyache that they get hours later. Thankfully, understanding parents can be there to help their children transition and have a relatively normal life, while still maintaining a gluten-free diet.

Involve the Whole Family

Children may need to maintain a gluten-free diet for a variety of reasons, including celiac disease, nonceliac gluten intolerance, or to help alleviate symptoms of autism or ADHD. Regardless of the reason, it's important to understand that this is a change that will affect the whole family, not just the affected child. Some families decide that if one person has to eat gluten-free, they will all eat gluten-free. This removes any temptations and possible conflicts that may arise by having foods that contain gluten in the house.

Other families decide to have a "shared kitchen," where both gluten and gluten-free coexist. Often in these cases, the family dinner is the one meal that is 100 percent gluten-free. This allows everyone to sit down and enjoy a meal together without anyone being treated differently. This arrangement is also much easier on the person preparing the meal, since the possibility of cross-contamination during meal preparation will be reduced or eliminated. With the "shared kitchen," meals that are less formal, or not attended by the entire family, may contain a mixture of gluten-free and regular foods. During these meals, cross contamination needs to be considered when preparing the food.

ALERT

Try to make both the gluten-free and the gluten-filled meals similar. If a child eating a regular diet is having cookies, have cookies for the gluten-free child as well. That way, everyone gets a treat and no one feels deprived while eating a gluten-free diet.

Remember, other than ensuring strict adherence to a gluten-free diet for the affected child, there are no formulas and no right answers for a family to follow. Experimentation and experience will help you figure out what works for your family and your budget. All family members should show care, concern, sensitivity, and patience as you work to develop a plan that's right for you.

Try to be considerate of anyone, children especially, who have to eat a gluten-free diet. Remember, the consequences of not maintaining the diet outweigh the loss of convenience. If a family works together to help a child maintain a gluten-free diet, the chances of that diet being successful increase greatly. It truly does take a village to raise a gluten-free child.

Get Some Help

Joining a support group is a great way to get additional help and support. You and your child are not alone; there are many children across the country, in your state, or even your city, who require a gluten-free diet to be healthy. Raising Our Celiac Kids (R.O.C.K.) is a support group designed to help families and friends deal with the changes and stresses that arise with a gluten-free diet. There are many chapters scattered across the United States. To find a chapter nearest you, or to find information on starting your own R.O.C.K. group, visit *www.celiac.com/articles/563/1/ROCK-Raising-Our-Celiac-Kids---National-Celiac-Disease-Support-Group/Page1.html.*

Talking to Your Child about the Diet

Once the shock of discovering that your child needs to eat a gluten-free diet has worn off, it's time to discuss this diet with your child. If your child is young enough, this conversation may be delayed until they are a bit older, since you will be providing them with all of the foods that they eat. Older kids, kids who are school age, need to have the new diet explained to them. Help your child understand that what they eat won't necessarily change, but it's where that food comes from that will change. For a child already accustomed to convenience or restaurant foods, foods that will now be off limits, the transition may be made easier by explaining that their favorite takeout pizza can be replaced with a homemade gluten-free pizza. Stopping at a drive-through for a burger on the way home, or ordering in pizza may not be possible anymore, but these foods do not have to disappear from their diet altogether. They just require special food now, food that is prepared without gluten. And with some research and preparation, you can find restaurants offering gluten-free so everyone can go out for a treat.

The importance of sticking to a gluten-free diet needs to be clearly explained to your child as well. They need to know that any amount of gluten can make them sick. If they sneak a cookie from a friend, or eat their sibling's crackers, they will get ill again, and it will take a while for them to get better. The reaction to ingesting gluten may not be immediate, but it will happen, and when it does, those cookies or crackers will not have been worth it.

FACT

If your children are old enough, have them help you read labels. Make a game of seeing if they can find products that are gluten-free. With new labeling laws coming into effect, more manufacturers are beginning to print "gluten-free" directly on the package.

Most kids know someone with an allergy. Schools are often nut-free because of serious nut allergies that exist among the students. And even though avoiding gluten is different from avoiding peanuts, comparing an intolerance to gluten to other food sensitivities is a great way to help a child understand and identify their dietary needs. Although some food sensitivities may subside with time, living gluten-free is not going to be a short-term diet if it is treating their celiac disease. Since it is not a diet that they will outgrow, explain to children that it is best to leave the gluten behind, and move on to a new gluten-free life.

Any change can be viewed as loss, and despite their natural optimism, children being put on a gluten-free diet may undergo various stages of grief.

- They can experience shock, where they can't understand how the body cannot tolerate something so commonly available in our society.
- They may experience emotional pain as they start a gluten-free diet, and realize all the things they can no longer eat.

- How this diet affects one's entire lifestyle, even as children, can be painful and frustrating. From there they may become angry. Adults may get upset when it takes twice as long to do the grocery shopping, because reading every single label takes time. Kids may get angry when they can't eat the cupcakes brought by a classmate.
- The next stage, regardless of age, is sorrow. A pity-party over the loss of convenience and favorite foods is common, especially since food doesn't just nourish us; it plays a large role in our social lives as well.
- Eventually something happens to turn that all around; we realize that the only way through these stages is to take control of the situation. It is at this point that those facing a gluten-free life begin educating themselves, learning all they can about gluten and where it can be found.

Begin keeping lists of safe foods and restaurants, and plan with your child and family how to handle the various situations you may face. The reward at the end of all this will be the beginning of a full, happy, gluten-free life. Helping children take control of their own situations takes the control away from gluten. Slipping back into sadness may happen at times, but it's important to help your child keep moving forward. These are all big changes for you and your child. It may be emotional at times, and for children, those emotions may express themselves in different ways. Watch for the various stages of grief, acknowledge it, but try to stay positive and encouraging. Talking to your child and walking through the transition process together will help them get through and embrace their new lifestyle while minimizing any associated pain.

Packing a Gluten-Free Lunch

One of the most difficult meals to prepare for a kid on a gluten-free diet is a school lunch. Recent improvements in commercially available gluten-free breads make packing lunch easier, but when your child is away from your supervision for meals, you need to trust them to maintain their diet. Packing a lunch that contains their favorite foods, whether that is an egg salad sandwich or a hot dog, and making sure their lunch is similar to their peers', will help them feel comfortable and blend in with the rest of the class.

By either baking or buying some gluten-free cookies, muffins, or cake, you can still pack a sweet snack in the lunchbox as well. Dried fruit or dried fruit snacks make a great sweet treat as well. Just be sure to read the labels to ensure that they have not come into contact with any gluten during the manufacturing process.

Nearly every traditional item that you purchase to send in your child's lunch can be substituted with a gluten-free alternative. Gluten-free granola bars, crackers, and pretzels are all readily available, and they all travel well in lunchboxes.

Don't forget about fruits and vegetables. Fresh fruits and vegetables are great to send along for a snack or lunch, and if your child enjoys fruit cups, they can continue to take those as well. By adding a small container of vegetable dip or hummus, your child may actually even enjoy eating their veggies at lunchtime.

Be sure to stress the importance of sticking to the gluten-free diet to your child and caution them against the time-honored tradition of trading sandwiches or muffins with classmates. Someone may want their wonderful lunch, which you packed with love, but that lunch is for your child only.

What to Tell Your Child's Teacher

A good teacher is one of the most important adults in a child's life, and can be one of the best advocates for a child with special needs while they are at school. This is true in cases of physical or mental disability, behavioral problems, or even intolerance to certain foods. But for your child's teachers to be their advocate, they first need to understand your child's situation fully. This will require that you educate them specifically about your child's gluten-free diet.

With luck, your child's teacher will already be familiar with celiac disease, nonceliac gluten sensitivity, or any other food intolerances. If not, start at the beginning and explain where gluten is commonly found—in all wheat, rye, barley, and oat products—and that it is dangerous for your child to eat. Mention that, although the reaction to gluten is not as quick as peanut allergies, it should be treated just as seriously. Emphasize that there is no such thing as a "safe amount" of gluten for your child to consume.

Look around the classroom and ask if any play dough, papier-mâché, fingerpaint, or other craft supplies might contain gluten. These items are common in preschool and elementary school classrooms. You may need to conduct the research yourself, but ask the teacher which brands of craft supplies are being used and let the school know if you find any problems. When necessary, offer to supply your child with a gluten-free version for classroom use.

Very often, there are special events in class that revolve around food—children's birthday parties, holidays, and class parties, to name a few. Ask the teacher to let you know when any events like this will be taking place so that you can be sure to pack an extra treat for your child to enjoy as well. Don't expect the other parents to be able to supply gluten-free treats for your child; take your child's needs into your own hands. If a birthday party is being celebrated, send along a gluten-free cupcake or cookie for your child to enjoy while the class is indulging in the supplied snack.

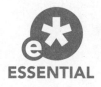

ESSENTIAL

Ask your child's school if it would be possible to store one or two treats in the staff room freezer for those instances when the class is having a special treat. Just in case a child brings cookies or cupcakes without the teacher knowing, your child will not be left out.

Discuss with your child whether to tell the whole class, only their close friends, or just the teacher about their gluten-free diet. There are benefits and problems with all three. Like most food intolerances, a gluten-free diet can't be kept a secret, and if the whole class knows, it may be easier to ensure that the diet is adhered to. Unfortunately, any special need may be used to taunt a child. Discussing the situation with your child, and their teacher, will help minimize this possibility and help you make the right choice for your child.

School Parties, Lunches, and Events

On days when you pack your child a standard lunch, it should be relatively easy to send them out the door with a gluten-free meal. But, there will be days when they have special parties or lunches that you may not have as much control over. The key to working through these food-related events is by communicating with the teacher and the school. Find out when these events are happening, and try to be prepared. You child may not be able to eat pizza or hot dogs during these events, but you can send along gluten-free pizza or hot dogs for your child to enjoy on those days. Once everyone is seated and busy eating, no one will care or even notice that one person's food didn't arrive with the food for the rest of the class.

If your child's class is having a special day of baking cookies or cupcake decorating, you can supply your teacher and child with the items they need so that they can participate too. For the cookies, send along prepared gluten-free cookie dough (cookie dough keeps very well wrapped in plastic wrap and refrigerated) and their own baking pan. This will ensure that they can participate in the activity as well. If the class is baking cupcakes and decorating them, send along baked gluten-free cupcakes and frosting that your child can use. By planning ahead, and having constant communication with your child's teacher, you can be prepared for nearly any food-related event that the class has.

Birthday Parties and Other Occasions

Every child (and adult) loves birthday parties! It is still possible to make a wish and blow out the candles while maintaining a gluten-free diet. If the birthday party is for your child or a family member, consider making all of the food gluten-free. By having all the treats, cake, ice cream, or candy gluten-free, the stress of knowing what is safe to eat is gone for one party. With great gluten-free recipes and commercial mixes readily available, it is possible to bake your child her favorite cake to help her celebrate another year.

If your child is going to be attending a party away from home, you will need to discuss the food with the person hosting the event. By finding out what is being served, you can determine if any of it is safe for your child to eat. You will also know what the other children at the party will be eating and, if necessary, you can prepare to send along similar foods for your child to eat at the party. If the kids are having pizza, you can send along a small gluten-free pizza that is safe for your child to eat. Although you will not always be able to match the food exactly, at least you can let your child eat something that will make him feel like part of the party.

FACT

For younger children, who may be unable to effectively communicate the need for a gluten-free diet, bracelets, tags, or labels may be the answer. You can find child-friendly bracelets, tags for lunchboxes and backpacks, and stickers that let you label food that is safe for your child to eat. Try one of these websites: *www.medicalert.org*, *www.n-styleid.com/children.html*, *www.hopepaige.com*, *www.allermates.com*, *www.statkids.com*, or *www.inchbug.com/allergyalerts.html*.

It is probably best to send food along for your child to enjoy while he is at a party. This will help reassure you that everything your child eats will be safe and gluten-free. It may not be possible for your child to participate in the birthday cake feast, but by sending along a gluten-free cupcake, he can still be included in the festivities. If cupcakes are too much work, you can also send along Marshmallow Pops as a fun treat. Marshmallow Pops are simply large marshmallows placed on a wooden stick. Dunk them in melted chocolate, and then dip them either in small candies, sprinkles, or chopped nuts. These treats will look so great the other children attending the party will wish that they could have some too, so be sure to send along a few extras. When you send your child, make sure the host is aware of their dietary needs. That way they can monitor what your child is eating, and you can be sure that your child's health will be protected.

CHAPTER 11

Breakfast Recipes

Raisin Bran Muffins

These healthy muffins are packed with nutrients.
If you can't find rice bran, feel free to substitute it with another ½ cup ground flaxseed.

INGREDIENTS | SERVES 12

½ cup ground flaxseed

½ cup rice bran

1 cup buttermilk

⅔ cup brown rice flour

¼ cup potato starch

2 tablespoons tapioca starch

1 teaspoon xanthan gum

1 teaspoon baking soda

1 teaspoon baking powder

½ teaspoon salt

2 tablespoons hemp seeds (optional)

⅓ cup oil

1 large egg

⅔ cup brown sugar

½ teaspoon vanilla extract

½ cup rehydrated raisins

Why It Is Important to Rehydrate

If you do not rehydrate dried fruit before using it in baking, the dried fruit will steal moisture from the batter, and leave you with dried-out muffins. To rehydrate dried fruit, place in a microwave-safe dish with just enough water to cover and microwave for 1 minute. Let fruit sit for an additional 5 minutes before draining off the excess water.

1. Grease a 12-cavity muffin tin or line with paper liners. Preheat oven to 375°F.

2. In a small mixing bowl, stir together the flaxseed, rice bran, and buttermilk. Let sit for 10 minutes (while you get everything else ready).

3. In a large mixing bowl, combine the brown rice flour, potato starch, tapioca starch, xanthan gum, baking soda, baking powder, salt, and hemp seeds (if using). Set aside.

4. In a medium bowl, beat together the oil, egg, brown sugar, and vanilla. Add the buttermilk/flaxseed mixture and stir well.

5. Stir buttermilk mixture into the dry ingredients, just until blended. Fold in the raisins and spoon batter into prepared pan.

6. Bake for 15–20 minutes, or until a toothpick inserted into the center of a muffin comes out clean.

7. Remove muffins from the oven and allow to sit for 5 minutes before removing from the muffin tin and placing on a wire cooling rack. Allow to cool completely before storing in an airtight container.

Lemon Poppy Seed Muffins

Although the glaze is optional, it really enhances the tangy citrus flavor of the muffins.

INGREDIENTS | SERVES 12

⅔ cup granulated sugar

Zest of one large lemon (or two small ones)

1 cup sorghum flour

½ cup brown rice flour

¼ cup tapioca starch

1 teaspoon xanthan gum

2 teaspoons baking powder

1 teaspoon baking soda

½ teaspoon salt

Juice of one large lemon (or two small) plus enough milk to make 1 cup

2 large eggs

1 teaspoon vanilla extract

½ cup butter, melted and cooled

2 tablespoons poppy seeds

½ cup granulated sugar

¼ cup lemon juice

1. Grease a 12-cavity muffin tin or line with paper liners. Preheat the oven to 375°F.

2. In a large bowl, use your hands to rub together the ⅔ cup granulated sugar and the lemon zest, until the sugar is damp and the mixture smells like lemon. Add the sorghum flour, brown rice flour, tapioca starch, xanthan gum, baking powder, baking soda, and salt. Whisk until evenly combined.

3. In a separate bowl, whisk together the lemon juice plus enough milk to make 1 cup, eggs, vanilla, and melted butter. Pour into the dry ingredients and mix until just combined. Stir in the poppy seeds.

4. Spoon the mixture into the prepared muffin tin. Bake in preheated oven for 18–20 minutes, or until golden brown and they spring back when gently touched.

5. While the muffins are baking, prepare the lemon glaze. In a small saucepan over medium-high heat, combine the ½ cup granulated sugar and ¼ cup lemon juice. Stir until it comes to a boil. Boil for 30 seconds before removing from heat. Set aside until the muffins are done.

6. Remove muffins from the oven and allow to sit for 5 minutes before removing from the muffin tin to a wire cooling rack. While the muffins are still warm, either brush the tops with the glaze, or dip the tops in the glaze. Allow to cool completely before storing in an airtight container.

Moist Chocolate Chip Banana Muffins

These muffins are soft, moist, and studded with chocolate chips.
They are perfect for a quick breakfast or snack, and are a great choice for kids' lunches as well.

INGREDIENTS | SERVES 15

1 cup sorghum flour

½ cup gluten-free oat flour

¼ cup tapioca starch

1 teaspoon xanthan gum

½ cup packed brown sugar

2 teaspoons baking powder

1 teaspoon baking soda

½ teaspoon salt

2 large eggs

⅓ cup oil

½ cup sour cream (or plain yogurt)

1 teaspoon vanilla extract

1 cup ripe bananas, mashed
  (approximately 2 medium bananas)

¾ cup gluten-free semisweet chocolate
  chips

Changing Things Up

To change things up a bit, you can add either ½ teaspoon of ground cinnamon or ground espresso powder to the batter. Adding ½ cup of chopped pecans or walnuts is another great option.

1. Grease a muffin tin or line with paper liners. Preheat the oven to 350°F.

2. In a large mixing bowl, combine the sorghum flour, oat flour, tapioca starch, xanthan gum, brown sugar, baking powder, baking soda, and salt. Set aside.

3. In a medium mixing bowl, whisk together the eggs, oil, sour cream, vanilla extract, and mashed bananas. Pour the wet ingredients into the dry ingredients, and stir just to combine. Fold in the chocolate chips.

4. Spoon the batter into the prepared muffin tin. Bake in preheated oven for 20–22 minutes, or until a toothpick inserted into the middle comes out clean.

5. Remove muffins from the oven and allow to sit for 5 minutes before removing from the muffin tin to a wire cooling rack. Cool completely before storing in an airtight container.

Pumpkin Cheesecake Muffins

These muffins are coffee-shop worthy. Even though you dollop the cream cheese mixture on top, it bakes down into the muffins slightly, making it a moist, flavorful muffin.

INGREDIENTS | SERVES 24

8 ounces cream cheese, softened

⅓ cup granulated sugar

2 cups brown rice flour

½ cup plus 1 tablespoon potato starch

⅓ cup plus 1 tablespoon tapioca starch

1½ teaspoons xanthan gum

3 teaspoons ground cinnamon

1½ teaspoons ground nutmeg

1 teaspoon ground ginger

1 teaspoon ground cloves

1 teaspoon salt

1 teaspoon baking soda

4 large eggs

1 cup granulated sugar

1 cup brown sugar

2 cups pumpkin purée (not pie filling)

½ cup oil

¾ cup applesauce

Chopped nuts (walnuts, pecans) or pumpkin seeds to top (optional)

1. Grease muffin tins or line with paper liners. Preheat the oven to 350°F.

2. In a small bowl, beat cream cheese and ⅓ cup granulated sugar until light. Set aside.

3. In a large bowl, combine flour and starches, xanthan gum, spices, salt, and baking soda. Set aside.

4. In a medium mixing bowl, combine the eggs, 1 cup granulated sugar, brown sugar, pumpkin purée, oil, and applesauce.

5. Pour wet ingredients into dry ingredients, stirring just until combined.

6. Fill muffin tins half full. Put 1–2 teaspoons cream cheese mixture in the middle, pressing down slightly.

7. Sprinkle with 1 teaspoon chopped nuts or pumpkin seeds.

8. Bake in preheated oven for 20–25 minutes, until a toothpick comes clean from the muffin part (do not touch the cream cheese; it is very hot!).

9. Let cool in pans for 5 minutes before removing to wire racks to cool completely. Once completely cool, refrigerate in an airtight container.

Baked Pumpkin Crunch Oatmeal

*Baked oatmeal is so easy to put together, smells amazing while baking,
and makes a great breakfast—even on the mornings you are short on time.
It can be baked ahead of time and simply reheated for a warm, satisfying breakfast.*

INGREDIENTS | SERVES 9

½ cup pumpkin purée (not pie filling)

1 large egg

⅓ cup maple syrup

1 teaspoon vanilla extract

⅔ cup milk

1 teaspoon ground cinnamon

½ teaspoon ground ginger

¼ teaspoon fresh ground nutmeg

½ teaspoon salt

2 cups certified gluten-free oats

1½ teaspoons baking powder

½ cup chopped pecans (optional)

1. Preheat oven to 350°F. Lightly grease an 8" × 8" square baking pan. Set aside.

2. In a large bowl, combine all ingredients.

3. Pour into lightly greased baking pan, and bake in preheated oven for 30–35 minutes. Let oatmeal sit for 5 minutes before serving. Topped with some ice cream or whipped cream, Baked Pumpkin Crunch Oatmeal also makes a great dessert.

Reasons to Eat Your (Gluten-Free) Oats

Not only does baked oatmeal taste great, it's also good for you! Oats help lower cholesterol, regulate blood sugar, are a great source of iron, and help keep you full for hours.

Milk and Oat Bars

These homemade breakfast bars use whole grains and nuts to make the perfect portable breakfast. Be sure to check that your oats, nuts, and dried fruit are all gluten-free.

INGREDIENTS | SERVES 12

1 (14-ounce) can sweetened condensed milk

2⅓ cups certified gluten-free old-fashioned oats

1 cup raw almonds

¾ cup unsweetened dried cherries, cranberries, or blueberries

¾ cup shredded unsweetened coconut

¼ teaspoon sea salt

¼ teaspoon ground ginger

1 teaspoon vanilla extract

1. Preheat oven to 250°F. Oil an 11" × 7" baking pan. Set aside.

2. In a medium saucepan, heat the condensed milk. Do not boil. Stir in the remaining ingredients.

3. Pour the mixture into the prepared pan. Flatten with the back of a spoon or spatula, making sure the mixture reaches all four corners of the pan.

4. Bake for 60–70 minutes or until the mixture looks dry but is not browned. The mixture should only be slightly sticky at this point. Remove the pan from the oven and place on a wire rack. Allow the mixture to cool completely in the pan. Slice into bars.

Cinnamon-Raisin French Toast

Serve with your favorite syrup or sprinkled with confectioners' sugar.

INGREDIENTS | SERVES 4

2 large eggs
⅓ cup milk
2 tablespoons butter, divided
8 slices gluten-free raisin bread
Syrup, optional
Confectioners' sugar, optional

1. In pie plate or large bowl, beat the eggs and milk with a whisk.

2. In large skillet, melt 1 tablespoon of the butter over medium heat.

3. Dip the slices of bread in the egg mixture, coating both sides.

4. Put 2–4 slices of bread into the heated skillet at a time, and cook 1–2 minutes on each side until golden brown. Continue with remaining butter and slices of bread.

Crepes

Crepes cook so quickly, they cannot be left unattended.
If you need to thin the batter out a bit, add an additional 2 tablespoons of milk.

INGREDIENTS | SERVES 4

1 cup brown rice flour

⅓ cup potato starch

3 tablespoons tapioca starch

½ teaspoon xanthan gum

1 tablespoon granulated sugar

½ teaspoon baking powder

½ teaspoon salt

2 cups milk

2 large eggs

2 tablespoons oil

½ teaspoon vanilla extract

For Those Avoiding Dairy

Milk helps these crepes brown, but if you are avoiding dairy, substitute water. The result will still taste great but will be a bit paler in color.

1. In a small bowl, whisk together the dry ingredients until combined.

2. In a larger bowl, whisk together the wet ingredients until combined.

3. Pour the dry ingredients into the wet ingredients, and whisk just until mixed. The batter may still appear slightly lumpy.

4. In a hot, lightly greased 10" frying pan (about medium-high heat), pour approximately ¾ cup of batter in the middle of the pan. Lift the pan and tilt it to distribute the batter over the entire pan. The batter should cover the entire bottom of the frying pan when you are done.

5. Once little holes and air bubbles begin forming in the top of the crepe, use a spatula to carefully flip it and brown the other side. Because they are so thin, crepes do not take long to cook.

6. You can top them with your favorite syrup or fresh fruit, sprinkle them with sugar, or use any other of the multitude of toppings available. Roll up and enjoy!

Yeasted Pancakes

Leftover pancakes also make a great bread substitute for sandwiches.

INGREDIENTS | SERVES 6

2½ cups brown rice flour

⅔ cup potato starch

½ cup tapioca starch

1 teaspoon xanthan gum

2 teaspoons rapid-rise yeast

2 teaspoons granulated sugar

1 teaspoon salt

3 cups warm milk (120–130°F)

2 large eggs, beaten

¼ cup butter or margarine, melted

Get a Jumpstart on Breakfast

The batter for these pancakes can be mixed the night before and kept in the refrigerator until morning. Place the batter in the fridge before giving it a chance to rise. To use the next day, remove the batter from the fridge and let it sit on the counter for 30–40 minutes.

1. In a large mixing bowl, combine the brown rice flour, potato starch, tapioca starch, xanthan gum, yeast, sugar, and salt. Stir to mix well. Set aside.

2. In a medium mixing bowl, whisk together the milk, eggs, and melted butter.

3. Add wet ingredients to dry ingredients, and beat for 2 minutes. Cover and let rise in a warm place until doubled in size, about 30 minutes.

4. Do not stir the batter before making your pancakes; that will release all the air bubbles that have been forming in the batter. Ladle about ½ cup of batter onto a lightly greased frying pan or griddle over medium-high heat. Flip pancakes over once bubbles form on the top of the pancakes. Cook until second side is golden brown. If the pancake is browning too fast, reduce the heat.

5. Repeat with the remaining batter.

6. Serve with maple syrup, fresh fruit, whipped cream, or any other favorite toppings.

Buttermilk Pancakes

If you do not have any buttermilk on hand, add 1 tablespoon of lemon juice to the milk, stir, and let sit for five minutes before using.

INGREDIENTS | SERVES 5

½ cup corn flour (not cornstarch)
½ cup brown rice flour
⅓ cup potato starch
2 tablespoons tapioca starch
½ teaspoon xanthan gum
1½ teaspoons baking powder
½ teaspoon baking soda
½ teaspoon salt
1¾ cups buttermilk
¼ cup oil
2 large eggs
1 teaspoon vanilla extract

1. In a large mixing bowl, whisk together all the dry ingredients until evenly mixed.

2. In a smaller mixing bowl, whisk together the wet ingredients.

3. Pour the wet ingredients into the dry ingredients, and stir just until mixed. It is all right if the batter still appears slightly lumpy.

4. Pour ½ cup batter onto a lightly greased frying pan or griddle over medium-high heat, making pancakes that are about 4"–5" wide. Flip pancakes over once bubbles form on the top of the pancakes. Cook until second side is golden brown. If the pancake is browning too fast, reduce the heat.

5. Repeat with the remaining batter.

Fluffy Waffles

Waffles are a versatile meal that can be eaten any time of day.
They are perfect for breakfast, brunch, supper, or dessert. They can be made ahead of time
and frozen, and reheated in either a toaster or oven when ready to serve.

INGREDIENTS | SERVES 5

1⅓ cups brown rice flour

½ cup potato starch

¼ cup tapioca starch

1 teaspoon xanthan gum

2 teaspoons baking powder

1 teaspoon baking soda

½ teaspoon salt

2 teaspoons granulated sugar

2 cups buttermilk

6 tablespoons oil

2 teaspoons vanilla extract

2 large eggs

Feeding a Crowd

To serve the whole family a delicious meal of waffles at the same time, you can keep the waffles hot and crisp by placing them in a 250°F oven until ready to serve.

1. Lightly oil your waffle iron and set to desired temperature. Allow to preheat while you prepare the batter.

2. In a large mixing bowl, whisk together the brown rice flour, potato starch, tapioca starch, xanthan gum, baking powder, baking soda, salt, and sugar.

3. In a small mixing bowl, whisk together the buttermilk, oil, vanilla, and eggs.

4. Pour the wet ingredients into the dry ingredients and stir just until mixed.

5. Cook on preheated waffle iron according to manufacturer's instructions.

Ultimate Pumpkin Waffles

The tastes of autumn and pumpkin pie don't have to be just for desserts anymore.
These waffles are full of pumpkin goodness and spices.
They are perfect when topped with some sweetened whipped cream or maple syrup.

INGREDIENTS | SERVES 8

½ cup light brown sugar
6 tablespoons cornstarch
1¾ cups brown rice flour
½ cup potato starch
⅓ cup tapioca starch
½ teaspoon xanthan gum
3 teaspoons baking powder
1 teaspoon salt
3½ teaspoons ground cinnamon
4 teaspoons ground ginger
½ teaspoon ground cloves
½ teaspoon ground nutmeg
4 large eggs
2 cups pumpkin purée (not pie filling)
2 cups milk
½ cup unsalted butter, melted

1. Lightly oil your waffle iron and set to desired temperature. Allow to preheat while you prepare the batter.

2. In a large bowl, combine the brown sugar and cornstarch. Whisk to combine. Add the remaining dry ingredients, and stir to combine.

3. Separate the eggs—place whites into the bowl of a stand mixer (if using) or bowl, and yolks into a medium-sized bowl.

4. Add the pumpkin purée and the milk to the egg yolks. Whisk to blend and set aside.

5. Beat egg whites until stiff peaks form. Set aside.

6. While whisking, pour melted butter into egg yolk/pumpkin/milk mixture.

7. Add the pumpkin mixture to the dry ingredients, mix until just combined. If they are still slightly lumpy, that is all right. The lumps will smooth out when the egg whites are added.

8. Place half the whipped egg whites in the pumpkin mixture, and fold in. Add the remaining egg whites, and fold in until no white remains.

9. Scoop batter onto hot waffle iron, and cook until done. It may take a little longer than normal waffles, due to the moisture that the pumpkin adds.

10. Serve warm waffles with sweetened whipped cream or maple syrup.

Broccoli and Cheese Quiche in a Potato Crust

This quiche can be served hot or cold. It can be made the day before, covered with foil, and reheated in a 300°F oven for 15–20 minutes.

INGREDIENTS | SERVES 8

3 cups shredded potatoes sprinkled with 1 teaspoon of salt

¼ cup shredded Parmesan cheese

½ teaspoon ground black pepper

½ teaspoon salt

1 tablespoon butter, melted

1 tablespoon butter

½ small onion, diced

2 cloves of garlic, minced

2 cups small broccoli florets

½ large red bell pepper, diced

5 large eggs

1 cup milk

1½ cups shredded Cheddar cheese

½ teaspoon salt

¼ teaspoon ground black pepper

Don't Like Broccoli?

If you are not a fan of broccoli, feel free to use a well-drained package of frozen, chopped spinach in its place.

1. Preheat oven to 425°F and grease a 10" pie plate. Set aside.

2. Let the shredded potatoes sit for 10 minutes before squeezing in a clean tea towel to remove all of the liquid (or, you can use frozen hash browns, defrost and squeeze all the water out). In a large bowl, stir together the dried potatoes, Parmesan cheese, ½ teaspoon black pepper, ½ teaspoon salt, and melted butter.

3. Press mixture into the bottom and up the sides of the greased pie plate. Try to make the layer of potatoes even, making sure there are no holes in the crust.

4. Bake crust in the preheated oven for 20 minutes, or until the potatoes begin to brown. Remove from oven and let sit for 5 minutes.

5. Turn oven temperature down to 350°F.

6. In a large frying pan, over medium heat, sauté the onion, garlic, broccoli, and red pepper in 1 tablespoon butter until the onion is transparent and the broccoli is bright green, about 5–8 minutes. Remove from heat.

7. In a large mixing bowl, whisk together the eggs, milk, cheese, ½ teaspoon salt, and ¼ teaspoon black pepper.

8. Spread broccoli mixture over the potato crust, so there is an even layer of vegetables.

9. Pour the egg mixture over the broccoli mixture, being sure that everything is distributed evenly throughout the quiche.

10. Bake in a 350°F oven for 30 minutes, or until golden brown on top and egg mixture is set. Allow to sit for 10 minutes before cutting.

Skillet Frittata

Cast-iron skillets work great for frittata making. They cook evenly and are oven-safe.

INGREDIENTS | SERVES 6

1 tablespoon butter

1 tablespoon olive oil

½ cup onion, diced

1 pound asparagus, chopped

¼ cup fresh or frozen peas

1 cup crumbled feta cheese

1 teaspoon dried oregano

1 teaspoon dried dill

1 teaspoon dried parsley

½ teaspoon dried basil

½ teaspoon salt

½ teaspoon ground black pepper

7 large eggs

Why Use Butter and Oil in the Same Recipe?

While it seems counterintuitive to use two different kinds of fats to grease a pan, there is a good reason. Butter cannot stand up to the same high heat as oil, but adds flavor oil cannot produce. When using the two together, you can cook at a higher temperature, and still get the great flavor that the butter adds.

1. Preheat oven to 325°F. Heat the butter and oil in a 12" cast iron skillet over medium heat. Sauté the onion, asparagus, and peas until the onions are soft.

2. Meanwhile, in a medium bowl, whisk together the feta, oregano, dill, parsley, basil, salt, pepper, and eggs.

3. Pour the egg mixture over the vegetables in the skillet. Tilt the skillet slightly to coat all of the ingredients with the egg mixture. Cook over medium heat until the eggs are just beginning to set.

4. Place skillet in the oven and bake for 10 minutes or until the mixture is cooked through and just beginning to brown.

5. Remove from the pan and slice. Serve immediately.

Cheesy Scrambled Eggs

Try combining several cheeses to create your own favorite cheesy eggs.

INGREDIENTS | SERVES 2

4 large eggs
¼ cup milk
½ teaspoon salt
Pinch of black pepper
¼ cup shredded cheese, any type
1 tablespoon butter

1. Crack the eggs into a small bowl. Whisk until they are light yellow and mixed well.

2. Add the milk, salt, pepper, and cheese to the eggs.

3. Melt the butter in a skillet over medium heat.

4. Pour egg mixture into the heated skillet and let it cook. As the eggs start to set, use a spatula to break them up and turn them over.

5. When eggs are cooked throughout and no longer runny, remove them from the skillet and serve.

Breakfast Burrito

Burritos are favorites for lunch and dinner. Why not try a breakfast variation?

INGREDIENTS | SERVES 1

1 teaspoon oil

1 large egg, beaten

1 (6") corn tortilla

1 tablespoon shredded Cheddar cheese

1½ teaspoons salsa

My Corn Tortilla Won't Bend

Corn tortillas stored in the fridge have a tendency to break if used cold. To make them roll nicely, either microwave between two damp paper towels for 30 seconds, or fry them for one minute per side in a lightly oiled pan over medium-high heat.

1. Heat oil in a small skillet over medium heat. Add egg and stir it while it is cooking. Once the egg is no longer wet, it is done.

2. Place scrambled egg in center of tortilla. Top with cheese and salsa. Roll up and eat.

3. If you want your cheese melted, you can heat the burrito with cheese in the microwave for about 15 seconds before topping with the salsa.

CHAPTER 12

Kid-Friendly Lunches and Snacks

Creamy Corn Chowder

This hearty soup makes a cozy meal on a cold day.

INGREDIENTS | SERVES 6

1 tablespoon oil

1 small onion, finely chopped

3 medium potatoes, peeled and chopped

2 cups water

½ teaspoon salt

¼ teaspoon black pepper

2 tablespoons cornstarch

2 (15-ounce) cans corn, drained

2 cups milk

2 tablespoons butter or margarine

Is It Done Yet?

To test potatoes for doneness, insert a fork into a few different cooked potatoes. If the fork goes in easily, they are done.

1. In a large saucepan, heat the oil over medium heat. Add the onion and cook for about 5 minutes, stirring frequently.

2. Add the potatoes, water, salt, and pepper.

3. Turn up the heat until the mixture begins to boil.

4. When the soup starts to boil, reduce it to a simmer, and continue to cook for about 20 minutes, or until the potatoes are tender.

5. In a separate bowl, mix the cornstarch with a little cold water to avoid clumps.

6. Add the corn, milk, and butter to the soup. Stir in the cornstarch to help thicken the soup.

7. Continue simmering for another 20 minutes, stirring occasionally.

8. Cool slightly before serving. Try your chowder with a salad and fruit for a complete meal.

Tasty Tomato Soup

The perfect side to a grilled cheese sandwich, but also great to pack for a hot lunch at school.

INGREDIENTS | SERVES 4

10–12 ripe tomatoes
1 tablespoon oil
½ cup onion, chopped
3 garlic cloves, minced
1¾ cups gluten-free vegetable broth
1 (6-ounce) can tomato paste
1 teaspoon dried basil

How to Peel Tomatoes

With a sharp knife, cut an "X" into the bottom of your tomato. Place tomatoes in boiling water for 30–60 seconds. Using a slotted spoon, remove them from the boiling water and place in a bowl of ice water. Once they have cooled a few minutes, the skins will peel right off.

1. Peel and chop the tomatoes, then place them in a large bowl and set them aside.

2. In a large saucepan, heat the oil over medium heat. Add the onion and garlic and cook for about 3 minutes, or until the onion is tender.

3. Add the tomatoes, cover the pan, and cook for about 5 minutes to soften the tomatoes.

4. Add the vegetable broth and tomato paste. Bring the mixture to a boil over high heat, and then reduce it to a simmer. Cover the pan and cook for another 10–15 minutes.

5. Pour the soup into a blender or food processor, 1 cup at a time. Do not overfill the blender. (If you put too much into the blender at once, the hot liquid will overflow when you turn it on.) Blend the mixture until it is smooth.

6. Pour blended soup into serving bowls to serve and sprinkle with basil. Continue with remaining portions. It may be helpful to prepare this soup in advance and transfer the blended soup to a new saucepan on the stove to keep warm.

Grilled Cheese and Tomato Sandwich

What's better than a warm and crispy grilled cheese sandwich?
Here's a slightly different spin on the old favorite that makes it more nutritious, too.

INGREDIENTS | SERVES 1

2 slices gluten-free bread
2 teaspoons butter
1 slice Cheddar cheese
1–2 thin slices of tomato

1. Spread the butter on one side of each slice of bread. Make a sandwich with the cheese and tomato between the two slices of bread, with the butter on the outside of the sandwich.

2. Place the sandwich in the skillet over medium heat and cook it for about 2 minutes on each side, until the cheese is melted and the bread becomes slightly browned and crispy.

Egg Salad

Egg salad can be used as a sandwich spread or as a dip with crackers. Either way, it tastes so good you'll be surprised how easy it is to make.

INGREDIENTS | SERVES 2

2 hard-boiled eggs

1 tablespoon mayonnaise

½ teaspoon celery salt

¼ teaspoon black pepper

Paprika, optional

1. Peel the shells from the hard-boiled eggs and rinse the eggs.

2. Place the eggs in a medium-sized bowl and mash with a fork or potato masher.

3. Add the mayonnaise, celery salt, and pepper. Mix well. If you'd like, you can sprinkle paprika over the top of the egg salad.

4. Spread the egg salad on gluten-free slices of bread for a sandwich or place in a small bowl to be used as a dip with gluten-free crackers.

Cheesiest Macaroni and Cheese

Giving up gluten also means giving up the macaroni and cheese from a box. This homemade version makes a comforting, warm meal, or a great cold lunch.

INGREDIENTS | SERVES 4

1 cup uncooked gluten-free elbow macaroni

2 tablespoons butter or margarine

1 tablespoon cornstarch

¼ teaspoon salt

¼ teaspoon pepper

¼ teaspoon dry mustard

¼ teaspoon gluten-free Worcestershire sauce

1 cup milk

1½ cups sharp Cheddar cheese, cubed or shredded

2 tablespoons crushed gluten-free corn flakes

1. Preheat the oven to 275°F.

2. Cook macaroni noodles in a large pot of water according to package directions. Drain in a colander.

3. Melt the butter in a large saucepan over medium heat. Reduce the heat to low. Add the cornstarch, salt, pepper, mustard, and Worcestershire sauce. Stir until smooth.

4. Add the milk and cheese. Continue stirring until the cheese melts and the sauce is creamy and smooth.

5. Stir the macaroni noodles into the cheese sauce.

6. Pour the mixture into a 2-quart casserole dish. Top with the crushed corn flakes.

7. Bake 30–40 minutes, or until the casserole is heated through and lightly browned. Let the casserole dish sit about 5–10 minutes before serving so the cheesy, creamy sauce has a chance to thicken.

Mini Pizza in a Flash

Making a mini pizza is about the quickest lunch you can make.
It doesn't require many ingredients, and it's easy to personalize it for your child's tastes.

INGREDIENTS | MAKES 2 MINI PIZZAS

1 gluten-free bagel, split in half

2 tablespoons pizza, spaghetti, or tomato sauce

¼ cup shredded mozzarella cheese

Meat or vegetable toppings, optional

1. Preheat the oven to 350°F.

2. Place the bagel halves on a cookie sheet. Spread the pizza sauce over each bagel half. Top with mozzarella cheese and other toppings.

3. Bake 5–8 minutes, or until the cheese is melted.

Mexican Quesadillas

*After trying quesadillas with just cheese, be adventurous
and add some refried beans, guacamole, or black olives.*

INGREDIENTS | SERVES 2

2 large corn tortillas

2 tablespoons shredded cheese, any
type

Sour cream or salsa, optional

1. Place one tortilla on a large plate and sprinkle with the shredded cheese. Top with the second tortilla.

2. Cook in the microwave for about 20–30 seconds, until the cheese is melted.

3. Cool slightly. Use a knife or pizza cutter to cut the tortilla into 6 wedges. Dip in sour cream or salsa, as desired.

Never-Enough Nachos

For a quick vegetarian version, try making this without the beef.
You can enjoy it as a snack with friends or even as an appetizer before a family meal.

INGREDIENTS | SERVES 8–10

1 pound lean ground beef
1 cup prepared salsa
1 medium tomato
4 green onions
½ cup lettuce
2 cups gluten-free tortilla chips
½ cup sour cream
1 cup shredded Cheddar cheese

1. Preheat the oven to 350°F.

2. In a large skillet, cook the ground beef for 8–10 minutes, until it is cooked throughout. Drain the ground beef, and then place it in a large bowl.

3. Add the salsa and mix well.

4. Chop the tomato and onion, and chop lettuce into small pieces. Place in separate small bowls.

5. In a 2-quart casserole, layer the ground beef and the other ingredients, starting at the bottom:

   - Gluten-free tortilla chips
   - Ground beef/salsa mixture
   - Sour cream
   - Tomatoes
   - Onions
   - Lettuce
   - Shredded cheese

6. Bake nachos in the preheated oven for 20–30 minutes, or until the cheese is completely melted.

Take-Along Trail Mix

Trail mix is so versatile you can create your own versions, too. Try adding some yogurt-covered raisins, dry gluten-free cereal, candy-coated chocolate, or even popcorn.

INGREDIENTS | SERVES 4

½ cup small gluten-free pretzel sticks or twists

½ cup raisins

½ cup peanuts

¼ cup sunflower seeds

¼ cup gluten-free chocolate chips

In a large bowl, combine all ingredients. Store in an airtight container or resealable plastic bag.

There's Gluten in That?

Always be sure to read the labels on dried fruit and nuts to ensure that the products have not come into contact with gluten during the manufacturing process.

Cinnamon Toasted Pumpkin Seeds

A twist on the classic, salted pumpkin seeds of yesteryear.

INGREDIENTS | SERVES 12

2 cups fresh pumpkin seeds

¼ cup sea salt

3 tablespoons olive oil

2 tablespoons ground cinnamon

1 teaspoon ground ginger

½ teaspoon ground cloves

¼ teaspoon ground allspice

Pumpkin Power!

Pumpkin seeds aren't just something to throw away prior to carving a jack-o'-lantern. Also known as pepitas, they are a low-calorie snack that is high in manganese, magnesium, iron, zinc, and protein. Omega-3 fatty acids, a healthy fat, are also found in pumpkin seeds.

1. Preheat oven to 350°F. Place the pumpkin seeds in a large pot. Fill halfway with water. Add salt. Bring to a boil. Boil for 10 minutes. Drain thoroughly.

2. Drizzle the seeds with olive oil, toss to coat. Sprinkle with spices. Toss again to distribute the spices.

3. Line a baking sheet with parchment paper. Arrange the seeds in a single layer. Bake for 15 minutes. Stir the seeds. Bake an additional 5 minutes or until they are toasted. Cool prior to serving.

Chewy Granola Bars

These granola bars are perfect to grab on the way out the door.
Make up a batch and you will never be stuck without something to snack on.

INGREDIENTS | SERVES 26

2 cups certified gluten-free quick-cook oats

¾ cup rice bran

¼ cup ground flaxseed

¼ cup slivered almonds

¼ cup uncooked quinoa

¼ cup shelled sunflowers

¼ cup sesame seeds

¼ cup flaked coconut

⅔ cup brown sugar

½ cup honey

4 tablespoons butter

½ teaspoon ground cinnamon

½ teaspoon salt

2 teaspoons vanilla extract

1 cup chopped dried fruit (cherries, cranberries, blueberries, apricots, etc.)

Change Things Up

Feel free to substitute for the dry ingredients, fruit, and nuts to suit your taste. Just be sure to substitute equal amounts so that the ratio of dry ingredients-to-syrup remains the same. If you add too many dry ingredients, the bars will not stick together, but if you have too few, the bars will be overly sticky.

1. Preheat oven to 400°F. Line a large rimmed baking sheet with foil.

2. Mix together all the dry ingredients (oats, bran, seeds, nuts, and coconut) on the baking sheet. Place in the oven and toast for 10–12 minutes, stirring every few minutes to prevent them from burning. As soon as the ingredients are toasted, remove the pan from the oven.

3. While the dry ingredients are toasting, line a 9" × 13" pan with parchment paper and spray lightly with cooking oil.

4. Place a small saucepan over medium-high heat and add the brown sugar, honey, butter, cinnamon, and salt. Bring the mixture to a strong boil for 2 minutes, stirring constantly. Turn off the heat and stir in vanilla.

5. Place the toasted ingredients in a large bowl, and stir in the dried fruit. Pour the hot liquids into the bowl and stir aggressively until all the ingredients are moist and well combined.

6. Using a wooden spoon, scrape the mixture onto the prepared baking sheet, pressing down to evenly spread out the mixture. Using a wet rubber spatula helps to keep the granola from sticking, allowing you to press the mixture down enough. Set the baking sheet aside and let the mixture cool for 2–3 hours until it is hardened.

7. Once the mixture is hard, remove it from the pan and turn the granola out onto a cutting board. Remove the parchment paper. Cut the granola into bars by pressing straight down with a long knife (don't saw or they will crumble). Cut approximately 26 bars, 1" × 5½".

8. Wrap the bars individually in plastic wrap, and store in an airtight container at room temperature for up to a week.

Perfect Popcorn

High in fiber, low in fat, popcorn is the perfect whole-grain snack.
Making it at home is a breeze. No microwave required!

INGREDIENTS | SERVES 4

3 tablespoon oil
⅓ cup popcorn kernels

Popcorn Suggestions

Popcorn can be flavored with nearly any-thing! If using air-popped popcorn, a driz-zle of butter will help the spices adhere. Some toppings to try are Parmesan cheese, popcorn salt and butter, chopped chives, chili powder, and lime zest.

1. Heat the oil in a 3-quart lidded saucepan. Test the temperature by tossing a few kernels in. If they pop, the oil is ready. Add the rest of the popcorn. Cover. Once the popcorn starts to pop, carefully shake the pan by sliding it back and forth over the burner.

2. Once the popcorn stops popping in earnest, and there are several seconds between pops, remove from heat and pour into a bowl. Add desired toppings.

Nutty Caramel Corn

A fun snack for the fall, this fan favorite is commonly seen around Halloween.
Try it along with some caramel apples, and you will have a party.

INGREDIENTS | SERVES 6

1 (3½-ounce) bag plain microwave popcorn, popped
1 cup dry-roasted, salted peanuts
1 cup brown sugar
½ cup butter
½ cup corn syrup
¼ teaspoon salt

1. Preheat the oven to 200°F. Spray a 9" × 13" baking pan with cooking spray.

2. In a large bowl, combine the popped popcorn and nuts.

3. In a medium saucepan, combine the brown sugar, butter, corn syrup, and salt.

4. Heat over medium-high heat until mixture is melted and smooth, stirring constantly. This should take 4–5 minutes.

5. Remove from heat and pour caramel mixture over the popcorn and nuts, mixing well. Spread out the popcorn mixture on the prepared baking pan.

6. Bake 1 hour, stirring every 15 minutes.

No-Bake Honey Balls

Let the kids get their hands dirty. These sweet and chewy no-bake cookies are a good choice for beginning cooks.

INGREDIENTS | SERVES 15

½ cup honey

½ cup golden raisins

½ cup dry milk powder

1 cup gluten-free crushed crisp rice cereal

¼ cup confectioners' sugar

1 cup finely chopped dates

1 cup gluten-free crushed crisp rice cereal

1. In a food processor, combine honey and raisins; process until smooth. Scrape into a small bowl and add milk powder, 1 cup crushed cereal, confectioners' sugar, and dates; mix well. You may need to add more powdered sugar or honey for desired consistency.

2. Form mixture into ¾" balls and roll in remaining crushed cereal. Store in airtight container at room temperature.

Dates

Do not buy the precut dates that have been coated in sugar for most recipes. They are too dry and too sweet and will upset the balance of most recipes. To chop dates, use scissors occasionally dipped into very hot water. If you can find them, Medjool dates, usually found in health food and gourmet stores, are richer than Deglet Noor dates.

Cinnamon Apples to Go

When you take these to go, remember to grab a napkin.
You will enjoy eating them so much, you will lick your fingers clean.

INGREDIENTS | SERVES 1

1 apple, any variety
1 teaspoon sugar
½ teaspoon cinnamon

That's a Lot of Apples!

There are more than 2,500 varieties of apples grown in the United States, and more than 100 varieties are produced commercially. On average, Americans eat about 50 pounds of apple products, per person, per year.

1. Peel apple. Remove seeds and cut into thin slices. Place apple slices into a small resealable plastic bag.

2. Measure sugar and cinnamon directly into bag over apple slices.

3. Shake your bag. Take your apple slices to go.

Best Banana-Berry Smoothie

You can enjoy this smoothie any time of year. It's delicious, refreshing, and good for you. And it's a great choice for breakfast on the go!

INGREDIENTS | SERVES 2

1 frozen banana

½ cup frozen berries (raspberries, blueberries, strawberries, or any combination you choose)

1 (8-ounce) container vanilla yogurt

½ cup milk

1. Put all the ingredients into a blender.

2. Put the lid on and blend for 1 minute, or until smooth. Pour into large glasses and enjoy.

Freezing a Banana

When a banana becomes too ripe and soft to eat, you can freeze it to keep on hand for smoothies and frozen beverages. Peel the banana and then wrap it up in plastic wrap and place it in the freezer; otherwise, you will have a hard time removing the peel.

Slushies

These brain-freezing flavored ice drinks are perfect to enjoy on those hot, humid summer days. No need to drive down to the nearest convenience store for these anymore—just make them at home!

INGREDIENTS | SERVES 4

1 package unsweetened Kool-Aid drink mix, any flavor

2 cups cold water

¼–½ cup granulated sugar

4 cups ice

1. In a blender, combine Kool-Aid, water, and sugar. Blend. Add all the ice and blend again.

2. Pour into cups, add a straw, and enjoy on those hot summer days.

Strawberry Granita

Fresh strawberries add flavor, fiber, and a beautiful pink color to this granita.

INGREDIENTS | SERVES 4

1 cup water

1 cup sugar

4 cups whole strawberries

What Is a Granita?

Originally from Sicily, granitas are a popular Italian treat. Similar to Italian ices, granitas are also made from sugar, water, and flavorings. Unlike Italian ices, however, they are made with flavored liquid, rather than plain ice simply doused with flavoring. Their texture should be flaky and granular, not too chunky or icy.

1. Bring the water and sugar to a boil in a medium saucepan. Boil, stirring occasionally, until it reduces and thickens into a light syrup. Remove from heat and allow to fully cool.

2. Pour the syrup into a blender. Add the strawberries. Pulse until smooth.

3. Pour the mixture into a 13" × 9" metal pan. Freeze for 20 minutes.

4. Remove from the freezer and rake any frozen bits with a fork. Return to the freezer for 20 additional minutes.

5. Remove from the freezer and rake any frozen bits with a fork. Freeze for an additional 30 minutes.

6. Remove from the freezer and rake again. Serve.

CHAPTER 13

Main Dish Recipes

Mexican Lasagna

Although this dish goes together quick enough for a weeknight meal,
you can also make the lasagna ahead of time and keep it covered in the refrigerator.
This will require you to increase the baking time by 20–30 minutes.

INGREDIENTS | SERVES 12

1¼ pounds lean ground beef
½ cup onion, diced
½ cup red pepper, diced
1½ cups frozen corn
1 (19-ounce) can kidney beans
2 tablespoons taco seasoning
1½ cups salsa
1 cup sour cream
15 (4") corn tortillas
3 cups Cheddar cheese, shredded
Chopped cilantro for garnish, optional

Make Your Own Taco Seasoning

Mix together 2 tablespoons chili powder, 2 teaspoons ground cumin, 1 teaspoon each paprika and salt, and ½ teaspoon each garlic powder, onion powder, dried oregano, and ground black pepper. Store in an airtight container, and use in any recipes that call for taco seasoning.

1. Grease one 9" × 13" pan, and preheat the oven to 375°F.

2. In a large skillet, cook the ground beef until nearly cooked. While it is still moist, add the chopped onion, red pepper, and corn. Fry, stirring occasionally, until the onion is transparent and the corn is defrosted.

3. Add the kidney beans, taco seasoning, and salsa and continue stirring to heat throughout. Stir in the sour cream and set aside.

4. Cut nine of the corn tortillas in half. This will allow you to have the tortilla layer going to the edge of your pan.

5. Line the bottom of your pan with 5 corn tortillas (6 halves and 2 whole), with the straight side of the halves facing the outside.

6. Top with half of the ground beef mixture.

7. Sprinkle on half of the cheese followed by another layer of corn tortillas.

8. Spread the remaining ground beef mixture over the lasagna.

9. Top with the third layer of corn tortillas and sprinkle with the remaining cheese.

10. Cover with foil and bake in preheated oven for 30 minutes. Allow to sit for 5 minutes before slicing and serving. Sprinkle with chopped cilantro before serving (optional).

Pot Roast

Few things are as comforting as the smell of a slow cooking pot roast.
Chop leftover roast for sandwiches during the week.

INGREDIENTS | SERVES 6

2–3 pound chuck roast

1 medium onion, cut into wedges

2 sticks celery, cut into large pieces

2–3 carrots, chopped

1 quart low-sodium, gluten-free beef broth

½ teaspoon ground black pepper

¾ teaspoon dried rosemary

½ teaspoon dried thyme

1 bay leaf

¼ cup cold water

¼ cup cornstarch

Salt and pepper, to taste

1. Place roast, onions, celery sticks, and carrots in a heavy casserole dish or stockpot with a tight fitting lid. Pour the beef broth over the roast and vegetables, and add in the pepper, rosemary, thyme, and bay leaf.

2. Cover and bake at 275°F for 3–4 hours. The roast will be done when a fork can easily be inserted into the roast, and the meat is fall-apart tender.

3. Remove roast from casserole to plate, and cover with foil. Let it sit for 10 minutes before cutting.

4. While the roast is resting, it is time to make the delicious gravy. Strain the remaining beef broth into a medium stockpot. This will remove the cooked vegetables and herbs. Bring the broth to a boil over medium-high heat. Whisk together the cold water and cornstarch. While the broth mixture is boiling, slowly whisk in *some* of the water/cornstarch mixture to thicken the gravy. Add only enough of the cornstarch mixture until you reach your desired consistency. Remember, gravy will always thicken a little bit more as it cools, so you still want your gravy to be slightly runny so that it is not thick when you serve it. Season your gravy with salt and pepper to your liking.

5. Using a sharp knife (or an electric knife), cut the roast across the grain, or across the muscle fibers. Cutting the meat this way will shorten the fibers, making your meat seem more tender.

Meatballs

*Make a batch or two of these meatballs and freeze them
to make your own submarine sandwiches, or add them to pasta sauce.*

INGREDIENTS | MAKES 18 MEATBALLS

1 tablespoon olive oil

½ cup finely minced onion

2 cloves garlic, minced

½ teaspoon dried basil

½ teaspoon dried oregano

½ teaspoon dried thyme

½ cup gluten-free beef stock

½ cup gluten-free crisp rice cereal or
   corn flakes, crushed

1¼ pounds extra-lean ground beef

1. Preheat oven to 350°F. In small saucepan, heat olive oil over medium heat. Add onion and garlic; cook and stir until tender, about 6 minutes. Place in large bowl and let cool for 10 minutes.

2. Add basil, oregano, thyme, beef stock, and crushed cereal; mix well. Add beef; mix gently but thoroughly with hands until combined. Form into 18 meatballs.

3. Place meatballs on a parchment lined cookie sheet that has sides. Bake 25–35 minutes, or until meatballs are browned and cooked through.

Freezing Meatballs

Meatballs freeze very well, before or after cooking. Make a batch or two to have on hand so you can have spaghetti and meatballs at a moment's notice. If cooked, cool the meatballs completely and freeze in a single layer on a cookie sheet. Pack in hard-sided freezer containers, label, seal, and freeze up to 6 months.

Sloppy Joes

Sloppy Joes are perfect for children's parties, as the meat can be kept in a slow cooker on low heat for hours before serving. Just be sure to add more water if it seems to be getting too dry.

INGREDIENTS | SERVES 8

2 pounds lean ground beef

1½ teaspoons onion powder

½ teaspoon garlic powder

1 tablespoon gluten-free Worcestershire sauce

½ cup ketchup

1 teaspoon chili powder

¼ cup brown sugar

¾ cup water

2 tablespoons white vinegar

1 tablespoon prepared yellow mustard

1 teaspoon salt

½ teaspoon ground black pepper

Gluten-free Buns (see recipe in Chapter 15)

1. In a large frying pan, cook the ground beef over medium heat until completely browned. To eliminate a lot of the fat, you can spoon the beef into a colander, and rinse under running hot water before returning it to the frying pan.

2. Add the rest of the ingredients. Bring to a boil, and then turn heat down to low and simmer for 20–30 minutes, stirring occasionally.

3. Serve on gluten-free Buns with your favorite toppings.

Great for Even the Pickiest Eaters

By using dried garlic and onion powder, this recipe is full of great flavor and perfect for those picky eaters who don't like to see chopped onions in their food. If you wish, you can use ½ cup diced onion and 1 clove minced garlic in place of the dried powders.

Lean Beef Stroganoff

This rich recipe is wonderful for entertaining. Serve with a salad and some gluten-free garlic bread.

INGREDIENTS | SERVES 6

2 tablespoons olive oil

2 tablespoons potato starch

½ cup milk

1 cup gluten-free beef stock

1 tablespoon lemon juice

1 pound sirloin steak

1 tablespoon potato starch

½ teaspoon salt

⅛ teaspoon ground black pepper

1 tablespoon olive oil

½ cup onion, chopped

3 cloves garlic, minced

1 (8-ounce) package sliced mushrooms

½ teaspoon dried thyme leaves

1 (12-ounce) package gluten-free rice noodles

1 tablespoon gluten-free Dijon mustard

Stroganoff

Beef Stroganoff is a dish from Russia that is typically made of steak or other beef cuts simmered in sour cream, served over noodles. Adding vegetables adds nutrition, texture, and flavor to this classic recipe.

1. Bring a large pot of water to a boil. Meanwhile, in a small saucepan heat 2 tablespoons of olive oil over medium heat. Add potato starch; cook and stir with a wire whisk until bubbly. Add milk, 1 cup beef stock, and lemon juice and bring to a simmer. Reduce heat to low and simmer 5 minutes, stirring frequently, until thick. Set aside.

2. Cut steak into ¼" × 4" strips. Toss with 1 tablespoon potato starch, salt, and pepper. In large skillet, heat 1 tablespoon olive oil over medium heat. Add steak; brown, stirring occasionally, 4–5 minutes. Add onion, garlic, mushrooms, and thyme; cook and stir 5–6 minutes.

3. Cook rice noodles as directed on package until al dente. Add stock mixture and mustard to steak mixture in skillet; simmer 5–6 minutes to blend flavors. When noodles are cooked, drain and add to skillet. Stir to coat noodles. Serve immediately.

Beef and Broccoli Stir-Fry

Ordering in Chinese food can be difficult when you are on a gluten-free diet. But, you can still make some of your favorite recipes at home, and it really doesn't take very long.

INGREDIENTS | SERVES 4

¼ cup water

¼ cup gluten-free soy sauce

2 cloves garlic, minced

¼ teaspoon ground black pepper

1 pound stir-fry beef (or boneless round steak, cut into thin 3" strips)

2 tablespoons oil

½ cup onion, chopped (or thinly sliced)

½ cup carrots, thinly sliced

4 cups broccoli florets

1 cup cold water

¼ cup gluten-free soy sauce

¼ cup brown sugar

1½ teaspoons ground ginger

1 teaspoon sesame oil

¼ teaspoon red pepper flakes (optional, adds some nice heat)

¼ cup cornstarch

1–2 teaspoons toasted sesame seeds

1. In a glass bowl, whisk together the ¼ cup water, ¼ cup soy sauce, minced garlic, and black pepper. Add the stir-fry beef strips and marinade for half an hour.

2. In a large frying pan or wok, heat the 2 tablespoons of oil over medium-high heat. Add the stir-fry beef and marinade, and fry until the meat is no longer pink, about 3–5 minutes.

3. Add the onions and carrots, and fry, while continuing to stir, for another 2 minutes. Add the broccoli and continue stirring and frying for an additional minute.

4. In a small bowl, whisk together the 1 cup cold water, ¼ cup soy sauce, brown sugar, ginger, sesame oil, red pepper flakes, and cornstarch. Pour this mixture over the beef and broccoli mixture, and cook until sauce thickens, about 2–3 more minutes.

5. Serve immediately over hot rice. Sprinkle with toasted sesame seeds before serving.

Chicken Stir-Fry

Use this simple, versatile recipe the next time you are craving Chinese takeout.
Feel free to alter the vegetables to incorporate your favorites.

INGREDIENTS | SERVES 6

4 (4-ounce) boneless, skinless chicken
  breasts
2 tablespoons gluten-free soy sauce
½ teaspoon ground ginger
¼ teaspoon garlic powder
3 tablespoons oil, divided
2 cups broccoli florets
1 cup bean sprouts
½ cup red pepper, diced
1 cup carrots, thinly sliced
1 small onion, chopped
1 clove garlic, minced
2 cups water
2 teaspoons gluten-free chicken bouillon
  granules
½ cup gluten-free soy sauce
3 tablespoons cornstarch

1. Cut chicken into ½" strips; place in a resealable plastic bag. Combine 2 tablespoons gluten-free soy sauce, ground ginger, and garlic powder. Add to bag and shake well. Let marinate in refrigerator for at least 30 minutes.

2. In a large skillet or wok, heat 1 tablespoon oil over medium-high heat. Add the chicken and marinade and stir-fry until the chicken is no longer pink, about 3–5 minutes. Remove from skillet and keep warm.

3. Add the remaining 2 tablespoons oil and stir-fry the broccoli, bean sprouts, red pepper, carrots, onion, and garlic for 4–5 minutes, or until crisp-tender. Return chicken to the wok.

4. In a large measuring cup, combine the water, chicken bouillon, ½ cup gluten-free soy sauce, and cornstarch. Pour into wok and continue stirring until the sauce thickens and is bubbly.

5. Serve over hot rice noodles or rice.

Baked Chicken Fingers

Be sure to make extra chicken fingers! Leftovers are a great addition to salads and wraps for a quick, satisfying lunch.

INGREDIENTS | SERVES 4

4 skinless, boneless chicken breasts

1 cup buttermilk

2 egg whites

2 tablespoons water

2 cups gluten-free corn flakes, crushed

1 tablespoon Parmesan cheese, shredded

½ teaspoon each paprika, cayenne pepper, salt, pepper, Italian seasoning, and garlic powder

Why the Buttermilk?

Soaking chicken in buttermilk before cooking or frying it makes it more tender. In addition to adding to the flavor of the meat, the acidity in the buttermilk also helps to break down the cellular walls of the chicken, giving you moist, tender chicken once it is cooked.

1. Preheat oven to 400°F.

2. Cut chicken breasts into thin strips. Soak in buttermilk for 30 minutes. Drain and discard the buttermilk.

3. In a shallow dish, mix egg whites and water. Set aside.

4. In another shallow dish, mix crushed corn flakes, Parmesan cheese, and spices. Set aside.

5. Dip drained chicken, one strip at a time, into egg/water mixture, then into crumb mixture, until totally coated. Place chicken strip on parchment lined baking sheet. Continue with the rest of the chicken.

6. Bake in preheated oven for 30–40 minutes, or until done (cooking time will vary based on the size of the chicken strips).

Penne with Pesto and Chicken

This dish is so delicious and quick to put together. It is good enough to serve company, but quick enough to make on a busy weeknight.

INGREDIENTS | SERVES 8

1 (16-ounce) package gluten-free penne pasta

2 tablespoons butter

2 tablespoons olive oil

4 skinless, boneless chicken breasts, cut into bite-sized pieces

2 cloves garlic, minced

¾ cup gluten-free chicken broth

¾ cup milk

1 tablespoon cornstarch

Salt and black pepper, to taste

⅓ cup basil pesto

½ cup grated Parmesan cheese, divided

1 cup broccoli florets

Change Things Up

This dish is very versatile. If you or your family do not like broccoli, simply substitute with either asparagus or peas; both work great in this dish. Use your favorite gluten-free pasta. Pasta made from rice, corn, or quinoa all work wonderfully.

1. Bring a large pot of slightly salted water to a boil. Add pasta and cook according to package directions, or until al dente. Drain and rinse pasta with hot water.

2. Heat butter and olive oil in a large skillet over medium heat. Sauté chicken and garlic until chicken is almost cooked.

3. In a small bowl, stir together chicken broth, milk, and cornstarch. Pour into skillet with chicken and garlic. Season to taste with salt and pepper.

4. Add pesto and half of the Parmesan cheese.

5. Add broccoli and cook until broccoli is tender. Stir in cooked pasta, toss to coat. Top with the remaining Parmesan cheese and serve.

Fettuccine Alfredo with Chicken

When dining out, ordering Italian food can be difficult when eating a gluten-free diet.
Here is a restaurant-quality recipe you can make at home.
Add a tossed salad and a slice of gluten-free garlic toast, and your dinner is complete.

INGREDIENTS | SERVES 4

2 tablespoons olive oil

2 boneless, skinless chicken breasts

8 ounces uncooked gluten-free
   fettuccine noodles

½ cup butter

2 cloves garlic, minced

1 cup heavy cream

1 cup grated Parmesan cheese

Salt and black pepper, to taste

1 tablespoon fresh parsley, chopped
   (optional)

1. Heat olive oil in a small skillet over medium-high heat. Cook chicken breasts until done, seasoning with salt and pepper.

2. Prepare gluten-free fettuccine according to package directions. Drain and set aside.

3. Add butter and minced garlic to the chicken. Once the butter has melted, add the heavy cream. Heat until the cream is starting to boil, and add the Parmesan cheese.

4. Reduce the heat to low and cook until the cheese is blended and the mixture begins to thicken.

5. Stir in the drained fettuccine, seasoning with salt and black pepper to taste. If desired, add fresh parsley before serving.

Cornmeal-Crusted Chicken

This is a wonderful, moist, and tender chicken that is great served with mashed potatoes or fries.

INGREDIENTS | SERVES 8

3 pounds whole chicken, with skin on, cut up

2 cups buttermilk

½ cup cornmeal

¼ cup brown rice flour

3 tablespoons cornstarch

1 teaspoon salt

1 teaspoon ground black pepper

1 teaspoon onion powder

½ teaspoon garlic powder

Make This Dairy-Free

You can make vegan buttermilk by adding 1 tablespoon lemon juice to 2 cups of soy or rice milk; let stand for 10 minutes, stir, and use.

1. Place chicken in a large glass baking dish and pour buttermilk over the chicken. Cover and refrigerate at least 8 hours.

2. When ready to bake, preheat oven to 375°F. Line a large baking sheet with heavy-duty foil and spray the foil with nonstick cooking spray; set aside.

3. In a shallow bowl, combine all remaining ingredients and mix well. Remove chicken from buttermilk; shake off excess (discard buttermilk). Dredge chicken in the cornmeal mixture to coat.

4. Place chicken, skin-side up, on prepared baking sheet. Bake 45–55 minutes, or until chicken is thoroughly cooked and coating is a deep golden brown. Let stand 5 minutes before serving.

Chicken and Bean Tacos

Read the package on the taco shells to be sure they are gluten-free.
Let your family assemble their own tacos so they can pick their own toppings.

INGREDIENTS | SERVES 8

2 boneless, skinless chicken breasts

½ teaspoon salt

⅛ teaspoon ground black pepper

1 tablespoon potato starch

2 tablespoons olive oil

1 tablespoon lemon juice

½ cup onion, chopped

½ yellow bell pepper, chopped

1 (15-ounce) can black beans, drained and rinsed

1 cup salsa

8 gluten-free corn taco shells

2 cups lettuce, shredded

1 cup tomatoes, chopped

½ cup sour cream

1 cup Cheddar cheese, shredded

1. Preheat oven to 350°F. Cut chicken into 1" cubes and sprinkle with salt, pepper, and potato starch. Heat olive oil in large skillet and add chicken and lemon juice. Cook and stir until almost cooked, about 4 minutes; remove from skillet.

2. Add onion and bell pepper to skillet; cook and stir 4–5 minutes, or until crisp-tender. Return chicken to skillet along with beans and salsa; bring to a simmer. Simmer until chicken is cooked, about 3–5 minutes longer.

3. Meanwhile, heat taco shells as directed on the package. When shells are hot, make tacos with chicken mixture, lettuce, tomatoes, sour cream, and cheese. Serve immediately.

Beer-Battered Fish

When it comes to deep-fried foods, most fryers in restaurants are contaminated with gluten. However, you can still treat yourself to the occasional deep-fried meal at home, like this restaurant-style Beer-Battered Fish.

INGREDIENTS | SERVES 8

Enough oil for deep-frying, about 2" in your pot/fryer

8 (4-ounce) cod or tilapia fillets

Salt and black pepper, to taste

1 cup brown rice flour

¼ cup plus 2 tablespoons potato starch

2 tablespoons tapioca starch

2 tablespoons garlic powder

2 tablespoons paprika

2 teaspoons salt

1–2 teaspoons ground black pepper

1 large egg, beaten

12 ounces gluten-free beer

1. Heat the oil in a heavy bottom pot or a deep fryer until 365°F. Rinse fish, pat dry, and season with salt and pepper. Whisk together the brown rice flour, potato starch, and tapioca starch and place ½ cup of the gluten-free flour mixture into a shallow dish. Lay fish fillets in ½ cup of the flour mixture, just to coat them on both sides. Shake off excess.

2. Combine the remaining gluten-free flour mixture, garlic powder, paprika, salt, and black pepper. Stir egg into dry ingredients. Gradually mix in beer until a thin batter is formed. You should be able to see the fish through the batter after it has been dipped.

3. Dip fish fillets into batter, then gently drop one at a time into hot oil. Fry fish, turning once, until both sides are a golden brown. Drain on paper towels, and serve while still warm.

Grilled Salmon

Salmon is marinated and then grilled to perfection with this delicious and easy recipe. Perfect served with roasted potatoes and steamed veggies.

INGREDIENTS | SERVES 4

¼ cup orange juice

1 tablespoon lemon juice

2 tablespoons olive oil

1 tablespoon gluten-free Dijon mustard

2 cloves garlic, minced

½ teaspoon dried dill weed

4 (6-ounce) salmon steaks

Salmon

Salmon is so good for you. It contains omega-3 fatty acids, an essential fatty acid that your body cannot make. The fats in salmon help lower the risk of heart disease, reduce cholesterol levels, and reduce blood-clotting ability, which can help prevent heart attacks.

1. In a 13" × 9" glass baking dish, combine orange juice, lemon juice, olive oil, Dijon mustard, garlic, and dill. Add salmon steaks; turn to coat. Cover and refrigerate 1–2 hours.

2. Prepare and preheat grill. Make sure grill is clean. Lightly oil the grill rack with vegetable oil. Add salmon and grill on medium heat for 9–12 minutes, turning once, until fish flakes easily when tested with a fork. Discard remaining marinade.

Homemade Bean and Vegetable Burgers

Homemade bean burgers are much better than their frozen store-bought counterpart, and you know these don't contain any extra fillers.

INGREDIENTS | SERVES 4

1 (15-ounce) can dark red kidney beans, drained

1 large Yukon Gold potato, cooked and cooled

⅓ cup cornmeal

⅓ cup fresh or defrosted frozen peas

2 tablespoons minced onion

¼ teaspoon ground chipotle

¼ teaspoon paprika

¼ teaspoon freshly ground black pepper

¼ teaspoon sea salt

2 tablespoons apple cider vinegar

2 tablespoons oil

1. In a medium bowl, mash the beans and potato together using a potato masher. Add the remaining ingredients. Mix and form into 4 patties.

2. Heat the oil in a skillet. Cook the burgers, flipping once, until cooked through and browned on both sides.

CHAPTER 14

Sides and Salads

Colorful Grilled Corn Salad

*Although this salad is great paired with beef, chicken, or fish,
it is also terrific just eaten with gluten-free tortilla chips.*

INGREDIENTS | SERVES 8

6 cobs of corn, shucked and cleaned

1 (19-ounce) can black beans, drained and rinsed

1 red pepper, chopped

½ cup diced red onion

½ cup chopped fresh cilantro

1 jalapeño pepper, finely diced (optional)

½ cup olive oil

½ cup red wine vinegar

2 tablespoons lime juice

1 tablespoon agave nectar or sugar

1 teaspoon salt

1 clove garlic, minced

½ teaspoon ground cumin

½ teaspoon ground black pepper

1 teaspoon chili powder

Dash of hot sauce

1. Grill cleaned corn over medium heat for 15–20 minutes, turning occasionally, until slightly blackened in areas. Allow to cool and cut off corn into a bowl. Add black beans, red pepper, red onion, cilantro, and jalapeño pepper.

2. In a small bowl, whisk to combine the olive oil, red wine vinegar, lime juice, agave nectar, salt, garlic, cumin, black pepper, chili powder, and hot sauce.

3. Pour over corn mixture and stir to coat.

4. Refrigerate for at least an hour, or until ready to serve.

Great for Parties and Potlucks

This salad is the perfect dish to bring to the next barbecue or potluck that you are invited to. The dish is not only gluten-free, but also free from dairy, peanuts, tree nuts, fish and shellfish, eggs, and soy.

Waldorf-Inspired Quinoa Salad

This salad is tasty, but also very healthy. It can be served as a side dish, dessert, or even breakfast!

INGREDIENTS | SERVES 6

1 cup water
1 cup apple juice
½ teaspoon ground cinnamon
1 cup quinoa, well rinsed and drained
1 large red apple, cored and diced
1 cup celery, chopped
½ cup dried cranberries
½ cup walnuts, chopped
1 cup vanilla yogurt

1. Place water, apple juice, cinnamon, and quinoa in medium saucepan and bring to a boil. Reduce heat and simmer for 15–20 minutes, or until the liquid is absorbed. Cool, cover, and refrigerate quinoa for at least 1 hour.

2. Add diced apple, celery, cranberries, and walnuts to cooled quinoa. Mix well. Fold in the yogurt. Refrigerate until ready to serve.

Greens and Fruit Salad

This salad dressing can be used on any tossed salad. Try it the next time you make a pasta salad.

INGREDIENTS | SERVES 4

4 cups mixed salad greens

2 cups baby spinach leaves

2 cups red grapes

1 orange, peeled and chopped

¼ cup orange juice

2 tablespoons honey

¼ cup olive oil

1 tablespoon gluten-free Dijon mustard

¼ teaspoon ground ginger

¼ teaspoon salt

⅛ teaspoon white pepper

1. In a serving bowl, toss together salad greens, spinach, grapes, and orange; set aside.

2. In a small jar with a screw-top lid, combine remaining ingredients. Seal lid and shake vigorously to blend salad dressing. Pour over the ingredients in serving bowl, toss lightly, and serve immediately.

Packaged Greens or Fresh?

For the freshest greens, pick those that have not been processed and packaged and are ready to use. There is less risk of cross-contamination, and you have control over exactly what is in your salad. Wash the greens by rinsing in cold water, then dry by rolling the leaves in a kitchen towel.

Garden Medley Salad

This salad can be served as is, or you can toss it with mixed greens or fresh spinach.
Cooked chicken or ham can be added to make this a main-dish salad.

INGREDIENTS | SERVES 4

1 cup sliced carrots

3 stalks celery, chopped

1 cup small cauliflower florets

¼ cup chopped green onion

1 yellow bell pepper, chopped

1 cup cherry tomatoes

1 cup chopped cucumber

⅓ cup gluten-free Italian salad dressing

In a medium bowl, combine all ingredients except salad dressing and toss to blend. Drizzle salad dressing over all; toss to coat. Serve immediately, or cover and chill 2–3 hours before serving to blend flavors.

Vegetables for Salads

Most vegetables can be used raw in salads, as long as they are sliced thinly or broken or cut into small pieces. If you'd like, you could blanch the vegetables before adding to the salad. Drop the prepared vegetables into boiling water for 30–40 seconds, then immediately plunge into ice water to stop the cooking.

Sweet Rainbow Coleslaw

Eating a "rainbow" of colorful foods allows you to enjoy a variety of good nutrition. All the different colors contribute different nutrients to your diet. You can make this up to one day ahead of time.

INGREDIENTS | SERVES 4

1 (16-ounce) package cut-up coleslaw
  mix with carrots
¼ cup chopped green pepper
¼ cup chopped red pepper
6 tablespoons white vinegar
¼ cup granulated sugar
3 tablespoons oil
2 tablespoons water

1. In a large bowl, combine coleslaw mix and chopped peppers.

2. In a small bowl, combine vinegar, sugar, oil, and water. Mix well.

3. Pour dressing over coleslaw and stir to mix well. Place in the refrigerator until ready to serve. Stir again before serving.

Sweetened Baby Carrots

Baby carrots are made from full-sized carrots, but they're peeled and cut into smaller pieces to be more appealing. You can enjoy them raw or cooked, like this recipe.

INGREDIENTS | SERVES 4

1 pound baby carrots

1 tablespoon butter or margarine

2 tablespoons brown sugar

1. In a large saucepan, combine the carrots and just enough water to cover them.

2. Put the saucepan over high heat until the water begins to boil.

3. Reduce the heat to medium and continue cooking until the carrots are slightly tender, about 15 minutes.

4. Using a colander, drain the carrots and return them to the saucepan.

5. Add the butter and brown sugar to the saucepan, stirring until the butter is melted and the carrots are well coated.

Strawberry Mango Salsa

This salsa has a sweet and spicy side to it. It is great served with grilled fish or chicken, but also satisfying eaten with corn chips.

INGREDIENTS | SERVES 6

1 mango, peeled and diced
2 cups strawberries, cut small
1 jalapeño pepper, finely diced
¼ cup chopped cilantro
1 tablespoon balsamic vinegar
1 tablespoon lime juice

1. In a bowl, mix together the mango, strawberries, jalapeño pepper, and cilantro.

2. Add the balsamic vinegar and lime juice, and stir to coat all the fruit with the juices.

3. Allow to chill for 30 minutes before serving. Stir again before serving.

Baked Mexican Rice Casserole

A quick and easy side dish you can get into the oven in just a few minutes.

INGREDIENTS | SERVES 4

1 (15-ounce) can black beans, drained and rinsed

¾ cup salsa

2 teaspoons chili powder

1 teaspoon cumin

½ cup corn kernels

2 cups cooked rice

½ cup grated Cheddar cheese

⅓ cup sliced black olives

1. Preheat oven to 350°F.

2. Combine the beans, salsa, chili powder, and cumin in a large pot over low heat, and partially mash beans with a large fork.

3. Remove from heat and stir in corn and rice. Transfer to a casserole dish.

4. Top with cheese and sliced olives and bake for 20 minutes.

Rice Pilaf

This side dish is perfect served alongside chicken, pork, or beef.

INGREDIENTS | SERVES 8

2 tablespoons olive oil

½ cup onion, chopped

3 cloves garlic, minced

½ cup chopped celery

2 cups uncooked long-grain rice

1 teaspoon salt

⅛ teaspoon black pepper

4 cups gluten-free vegetable broth

2 tablespoons butter

Cooking Rice

For best results in cooking rice, first sauté the rice in a bit of oil until opaque. Then add water or broth, bring quickly to a boil, reduce heat, and cover. Don't uncover the rice as it cooks; just check it at the end of cooking time. Let the rice stand for a few minutes after cooking for fluffier rice with separate grains.

1. In heavy saucepan, combine olive oil, onion, garlic, and celery. Cook and stir over medium heat until crisp-tender, about 5 minutes.

2. Add rice; cook and stir 2 minutes longer. Sprinkle with salt and pepper and add broth.

3. Bring to a boil, then reduce heat to low, cover saucepan, and cook 15–20 minutes, or until rice is tender and broth is absorbed. Remove from heat; add butter and let stand covered for 5 minutes. Fluff pilaf with fork and serve.

Fried Rice

Fried rice doesn't have to contain egg! If you add some chicken or ham to this easy recipe, you've created a main dish.

INGREDIENTS | SERVES 6

¼ cup gluten-free vegetable broth

1 tablespoon gluten-free soy sauce

1 tablespoon minced fresh gingerroot

⅛ teaspoon ground black pepper

2 tablespoons olive oil

½ cup chopped onion

3 cloves garlic, minced

½ cup shredded carrot

½ cup chopped green onions

4 cups long-grain rice, cooked and cooled

1. In small bowl, combine broth, soy sauce, gingerroot, and pepper. Mix well and set aside.

2. In wok or large skillet, heat olive oil over medium-high heat. Add onion and garlic; stir-fry 3 minutes. Add carrot and green onion; stir-fry 2–3 minutes longer.

3. Add rice; stir-fry until rice is hot and grains are separate, about 4–5 minutes. Stir broth mixture and add to wok; stir-fry until mixture bubbles, about 3–4 minutes. Serve immediately.

Try a Rice Cooker

If you have trouble cooking rice, get a rice cooker. This inexpensive appliance cooks rice to fluffy perfection every time. Another option is to cook rice like you cook pasta—in a large pot of boiling water. Keep tasting the rice; when it's tender, thoroughly drain and use in a recipe or serve.

Twice-Baked Greek Potatoes

Potatoes always make a great side dish, but when you can give them some flair, they really stand out at the meal. These Twice-Baked Greek Potatoes take on the traditional flavors of Greece, by using spices like oregano, thyme, and basil, topped with feta cheese.

INGREDIENTS | SERVES 4

4 large russet potatoes, baked

1 cup crumbled feta cheese

1 cup sour cream (or plain yogurt)

½ teaspoon ground black pepper

1 teaspoon dried oregano

1 teaspoon dried thyme

½ teaspoon dried basil

2 cloves garlic, minced (or ¾ teaspoon garlic powder)

1 medium tomato, chopped

¼ cup chopped black olives (optional)

¼ cup chopped green onion

How to Bake Potatoes

You can wrap washed and dried potatoes in foil and bake in a 400°F oven until a knife can easily be poked into the potato, or about 1 hour. Or, you can bake them in the slow cooker with 2 tablespoons of water on low heat for 8–10 hours. Both methods will give you potatoes that are tender when a knife is inserted, and they are then ready to spoon out and season.

1. Let hot, baked potatoes sit for about 15 minutes before handling. Carefully cut about 1" off the top of the potatoes lengthwise. Scoop the potato out of the skin into a large mixing bowl, leaving the skins intact. Line the scooped out potato skins in a single layer on a baking dish.

2. Add the feta cheese, sour cream, pepper, herbs, and garlic to the potatoes, and mash using a potato masher until smooth. Stir in the tomato, chopped olives, and green onions. Spoon filling back into potato shells, until they are nicely rounded on the tops. If you have leftover filling, spoon it into a ramekin dish.

3. Place potatoes in preheated 400°F oven and bake for 15–20 minutes, or until heated throughout. Serve immediately.

Pesto Potatoes

This flavorful side dish is delicious served with a steak or some grilled chicken or fish.

INGREDIENTS | SERVES 8

4 pounds russet potatoes
2 tablespoons olive oil
1 small yellow onion, chopped
3 cloves garlic, minced
½ cup basil pesto
¼ cup plain yogurt

Make Your Own Basil Pesto

In a food processor, grind together 1½ cups packed fresh basil leaves, 1 cup packed baby spinach leaves, 3 cloves garlic, 2 tablespoons lemon juice, ½ teaspoon salt, and ⅛ teaspoon pepper. With motor running, add ½–¾ cup olive oil, until desired consistency is reached. By hand, stir in ¼ cup Parmesan cheese and 2 tablespoons water, if needed. Store tightly covered in refrigerator up to 3 days. Freeze for longer storage.

1. Preheat oven to 400°F. Scrub potatoes and cut into 1" pieces.

2. In a large roasting pan, combine potatoes with olive oil, onion, and garlic. Roast for 30 minutes, and then turn with a spatula. Roast 30–40 minutes longer, or until potatoes are tender and turning brown on the edges.

3. In a serving bowl, combine pesto and yogurt and mix well. Add the hot potato mixture and toss to coat. Serve immediately.

Parmesan Potato Fries

You can prepare these potatoes with or without the skin in whatever shape you like. Before you know it, they'll be a favorite at your dinner table.

INGREDIENTS | SERVES 4

4 russet potatoes
2 tablespoons oil
1 teaspoon salt
½ teaspoon pepper
1 tablespoon Parmesan cheese

1. Preheat the oven to 350°F. Line a baking pan or cookie sheet with parchment paper. Wash the potatoes. Cut them into strips or rounds or any shape you choose.

2. Put the potatoes into a resealable bag or a large bowl. Add the oil to the bag or bowl and mix until the potatoes are well coated. Sprinkle the potatoes with salt, pepper, and Parmesan cheese. Toss again.

3. Place the potatoes in a single layer onto prepared baking pan or cookie sheet. Bake potatoes for 45–50 minutes or until they are crispy and golden brown. Halfway through baking, flip over the potatoes so they cook evenly on all sides.

Smashed Potatoes

These rustic potatoes aren't mashed perfectly smooth.
The skins are left on, which adds nutrients and fiber.

INGREDIENTS | SERVES 6

6 Yukon Gold potatoes

3 tablespoons olive oil

3 garlic cloves, minced

2 shallots, minced

1 (3-ounce) package cream cheese, softened

2–4 tablespoons milk

½ teaspoon salt

⅛ teaspoon black pepper

1. Scrub potatoes and cut into 1" pieces. Bring a large pot of water to a boil. Add potatoes; bring back to a simmer. Simmer 10–20 minutes, or until potatoes are tender when pierced with a fork. Drain, and then return potatoes to the hot pot.

2. Meanwhile, in a small saucepan, heat olive oil over medium heat; sauté garlic and shallots for 2–3 minutes. Place pot with hot potatoes over medium heat and, using a fork or potato masher, mash in the garlic mixture. Leave some pieces of the potatoes whole.

3. Stir in the cream cheese, 2 tablespoons milk, salt, and pepper; add more milk if necessary for desired consistency. Serve immediately. Or you can keep these potatoes warm in a double boiler over simmering water for about an hour.

Hash Brown Casserole

This recipe makes a huge amount, so it's perfect for entertaining or holidays.

INGREDIENTS | SERVES 8–10

1 (32-ounce) package frozen hash browns, thawed

½ cup minced onion

2 cloves garlic, minced

1 teaspoon salt

¼ teaspoon ground black pepper

1 cup cream cheese, softened

⅓ cup milk

2 cups shredded mozzarella cheese

1. Preheat oven to 375°F. Spray a 13" × 9" baking dish with nonstick cooking spray and set aside.

2. In a large bowl, combine all ingredients and mix well. Spoon into baking dish and spread into an even layer. Cover and bake for 30 minutes, then uncover and bake 30–40 minutes longer, or until casserole is bubbly and starting to brown. Serve immediately.

Hash Browns

You can find hash browns in the refrigerated and freezer sections of your local grocery store. Read labels carefully, as some brands do contain gluten. To thaw the frozen potatoes, just let the bag stand in the refrigerator overnight. Drain the potatoes well before using in recipes.

CHAPTER 15

Breads

Fluffy Buttermilk Biscuits

These fluffy, light biscuits are perfect topped with jam and a slice of cheese. Or they can be used to dip in your favorite soup. Either way, it's a very versatile recipe that is sure to be used over and over again.

INGREDIENTS | SERVES 9

1¼ cups brown rice flour

¼ cup tapioca starch

4 teaspoons xanthan gum

2 teaspoons baking powder

1 teaspoon baking soda

½ teaspoon salt

1 teaspoon granulated sugar

½ cup cold butter, cut into chunks

2 large eggs

⅓ cup buttermilk

Milk for brushing the tops of biscuits before baking, optional

Coarse salt, optional

Make Savory Biscuits

To make these biscuits savory, you can add ½ teaspoon of garlic powder or Italian seasoning (or even both) to the dry ingredients. Another great add-in is 1 tablespoon fresh chopped chives.

1. Preheat oven to 425°F. Line a baking sheet with parchment paper, and sprinkle with some brown rice flour. Set aside.

2. In the bowl of a food processor, combine all the dry ingredients, and pulse to combine. (If you don't have a food processor, combine all dry ingredients in a medium-sized mixing bowl.)

3. Add the butter and pulse until the butter is the size of a lentil/pea. (Or, use a pastry blender to cut the butter into the dry ingredients, being sure to work quickly, because you want the butter to stay cold.)

4. Add the eggs and buttermilk, and run the food processor until the dough comes together in a ball. (Alternately, you can use a wooden spoon and stir until the dough comes together.)

5. Turn dough out onto the parchment-lined baking sheet, and flour your hands with more brown rice flour. Working quickly, pat the dough down into a square shape, approximately 10" × 10", and ¾" thick. Using a sharp knife, cut the dough into 9 biscuits.

6. Gently rearrange the biscuits so they are not touching and have room to expand while they are baking. Gently brush the tops of the biscuits with milk, and sprinkle with coarse salt (optional).

7. Bake in preheated oven for 14–16 minutes, or until golden brown. Allow to cool for 5 minutes on a cooling rack before serving. You can store the remaining biscuits in an airtight container.

Corn Bread Muffins

These muffins are perfect served with a piping hot bowl of chili, or eaten as a sweet treat topped with some fresh honey. Depending on how sweet you like it, you can cut the sugar down to ⅓ cup and still have great results.

INGREDIENTS | SERVES 12

½ cup butter or margarine

⅔ cup granulated sugar (or ⅓ cup if you prefer less sweet muffins)

2 large eggs

1 cup buttermilk

½ teaspoon baking soda

1 cup cornmeal

⅔ cup brown rice flour

3 tablespoons potato starch

2 tablespoons tapioca starch

½ teaspoon xanthan gum

½ teaspoon salt

1. Preheat oven to 350°F. Lightly grease a muffin pan and set aside.

2. In a large microwave-safe bowl, melt butter. Stir in the sugar. Add eggs and stir to combine. Stir in buttermilk.

3. In a medium-sized mixing bowl, whisk the remaining ingredients. Add to wet ingredients, and stir until few lumps remain.

4. Scoop batter into prepared muffin tin.

5. Bake for 20 minutes in preheated oven, or until a toothpick inserted into the center comes out clean.

6. Allow to cool in the muffin pan for 5 minutes before removing to cooling rack. Best served warm.

Bagels

This recipe makes 4 jumbo-sized bagels, or you can make 8 smaller ones. To freeze them, wrap them in plastic wrap and put them in a resealable plastic bag before putting them in the freezer. For that "just baked" feel, microwave them for a few seconds before eating them.

INGREDIENTS | SERVES 4

1 cup brown rice flour

½ cup sorghum flour

½ cup potato starch

½ cup tapioca starch

½ cup ground flaxseed

1 tablespoon xanthan gum

1½ teaspoons salt

1 tablespoon rapid-rise yeast

2 tablespoons agave nectar or honey

1 teaspoon apple cider vinegar

2 tablespoons oil

1¼ cups warm water

Large pot, ¾ full of water

1 tablespoon molasses

2 teaspoons vegetable shortening, to grease your hands to form the bagels

Optional toppings: sesame seeds, flaxseed, chia seeds, onion flakes, poppy seeds, or coarse salt

1. Line a baking sheet with parchment paper.

2. In the bowl of a stand mixer, mix all the dry ingredients together until well blended.

3. In a small bowl, whisk together the wet ingredients.

4. With the mixer slowly running, pour in the wet ingredients. Then mix on medium speed for 3 minutes.

5. Grease your hands with the vegetable shortening. Take ¼ of the dough, and form it into a bagel shape, being sure to use your finger to create a large hole in the center of the bagel. Place the formed bagels on the parchment-lined baking sheet. Give them a lot of space as they will grow a lot as they rise. Repeat to create 4 large bagels.

6. Place the baking sheet in a warm, draft-free place, and allow bagels to rise for 35–40 minutes, or until they are nearly doubled in size.

7. While the bagels are rising, fill a large pot ¾ full with water. Bring to a rolling boil, and add the molasses to the water. The molasses will create a nice chewy outside to the bagel.

8. Preheat the oven to 400°F.

9. When the bagels have finished rising, gently place one at a time in the boiling water. Boil on one side for 30 seconds, flip, and boil for another 30 seconds. Remove bagels from water with a slotted spoon, and place on a cooling rack that has been placed over another baking sheet, allowing the water to drip off.

Bagels (continued)

More on Flaxseed

Ground flaxseed is a great topping for these bagels—it contains fiber and healthy omega-3 fatty acids, and adds stability and texture to gluten-free baked breads. You can grind whole flaxseeds using a coffee grinder. Store ground flaxseed in the fridge or freezer, so it doesn't go rancid quickly.

10. Place boiled bagels back on the parchment-lined baking sheet. At this time, you can sprinkle the tops with whatever toppings you desire.

11. Bake the bagels in preheated oven for 20–25 minutes, or until they are a nice golden brown. Remove from oven, and allow to cool on a cooling rack for 10 minutes before eating. You can eat the bagels warm, or allow them to cool completely before storing in a resealable bag.

Oatmeal Cinnamon Raisin Bread

Toasted and topped with butter, cinnamon, and sugar, this bread is sure to be a hit at the breakfast table. Or, fancy things up a bit and use it to make some French toast.

INGREDIENTS | SERVES 12

½ cup certified gluten-free quick-cook oats

1 cup raisins

Hot water, enough to cover oats and raisins

¾–1 cup warm water (start with ¾ cup and add up to ¼ cup if necessary)

2 tablespoons granulated sugar

1 tablespoon instant yeast

2 teaspoons apple cider vinegar

2 tablespoons vegetable oil

2 large eggs

2 egg whites

1 cup brown rice flour

½ cup potato starch

½ cup tapioca starch

¼ cup dry milk powder

2 teaspoons ground cinnamon

2½ teaspoons xanthan gum

1 teaspoon salt

Why Apple Cider Vinegar?

Apple cider vinegar is used in a lot of gluten-free bread recipes. It helps give a greater rise, and more tender crumb, to the bread by acting as a dough enhancer, increasing the amount of ascorbic acid in the dough.

1. Place oats and raisins in a bowl and cover with hot water. Set aside and let soak for 10 minutes. Drain water using a sieve or strainer.

2. In a small bowl, combine warm water, sugar, and yeast. Stir and let sit until foamy on top. Then add the cider vinegar, vegetable oil, eggs, and egg whites.

3. Combine all dry ingredients together in the bowl of a stand mixer until well mixed.

4. Add the soaked oats and raisins to the dry ingredients. Turn the mixer (with the paddle attachment) on low speed, and slowly add the wet ingredients. Once combined, scrape down the sides of the bowl with a rubber spatula. Turn the mixer on medium and beat for 3 minutes.

5. Spoon the dough into a greased 9" × 5" bread pan. Let rise, uncovered, in a warm, draft-free place for 25 minutes or until it has reached the top of the bread pan.

6. Place bread in preheated 350°F oven, and bake for 30–35 minutes, or until nicely browned and the loaf sounds hollow when tapped on the top.

7. Remove loaf from oven, and leave in the bread pan for 5 minutes. Remove from pan and cool on wire cooling rack. When the loaf is completely cool, store it in an airtight bag. It can be left on the counter for 3 days, or frozen (wrap in additional plastic wrap if freezing).

Buns

Being able to eat food on a bun is definitely taken for granted while eating a regular diet. Bake a batch of these buns and you can eat your Sloppy Joes (see Chapter 13), burgers, and sandwiches on a bun again!

INGREDIENTS | SERVES 6

½ cup warm water

1 teaspoon rapid-rise yeast

1 teaspoon granulated sugar or honey

¼ cup plus 2 tablespoons brown rice flour

¼ cup sorghum flour

¼ cup potato starch

¼ cup ground flaxseed

2 tablespoons tapioca starch

1½ teaspoons xanthan gum

½ teaspoon salt

1 teaspoon apple cider vinegar

1 large egg plus 1 egg white

2 tablespoons oil

Thinking Outside the Pan

When it comes to gluten-free baking, sometimes you have to think of things a little differently. Since gluten-free buns need more support than wheat-based buns, you can't just form them on a baking sheet like you would regular buns. Repurposing 4" potpie tins for baking buns works great, giving you a nice sized bun for a burger. You can also use English muffin rings, jumbo muffin tins, or tins from canned tuna that have been washed really well.

1. In a small bowl, combine the warm water, yeast, and sugar. Allow to sit for 10 minutes, or until it gets nice and bubbly.

2. In the bowl of a stand mixer, mix together the brown rice flour, sorghum flour, potato starch, ground flaxseed, tapioca starch, xanthan gum, and salt.

3. Add the apple cider vinegar, egg, egg white, and oil to the yeast mixture. Whisk to combine.

4. With the mixer on low speed, pour the wet ingredients into the dry ingredients. Increase the mixer speed to medium-high and mix for 3 minutes, scraping down the bowl if necessary.

5. Lightly grease six 4" potpie tins and place them on a baking sheet. Divide the dough between the six tins, with each tin having about ¼ cup dough. Using a spoon dipped in water, smooth the dough into an even layer across the bottom of the tin.

6. Let dough rise in a warm, draft-free place for 20–30 minutes, or until the dough has nearly doubled in size.

7. While the dough is rising, preheat the oven to 350°F. Once the buns have risen, place baking sheet with the tins on it into preheated oven. Bake for 25–30 minutes. Remove from oven and leave in the tins for 5 minutes before removing buns to a wire cooling rack. Let cool before serving. Once they are cooled they can be stored in an airtight container.

8. Buns can be wrapped in plastic wrap and stored in a resealable bag in the freezer. That way you can remove the buns from the freezer as you need them.

Focaccia Bread

*You can use this bread as the basis for homemade pizza or top it with
fresh vegetables and cut in small squares for an appetizer.*

INGREDIENTS | SERVES 8

1½ cups white rice flour

½ cup millet flour

⅓ cup tapioca starch

1 teaspoon xanthan gum

1 tablespoon rapid rise yeast

¼ teaspoon salt

2 teaspoons granulated sugar

½ teaspoon apple cider vinegar

1⅓ cups warm water

4 tablespoons olive oil, divided

2 tablespoons cornmeal

½ teaspoon coarse salt

1 teaspoon dried thyme leaves

1. In a large bowl, combine flours, tapioca starch, xanthan gum, yeast, salt, and sugar; mix well.

2. Add vinegar, water, and 3 tablespoons olive oil; beat with mixer for 2 minutes.

3. Line a 10" springform pan with parchment paper and sprinkle the bottom with cornmeal. Spoon the dough onto the paper; drizzle with remaining 1 tablespoon olive oil and sprinkle with coarse salt and thyme.

4. Let rise for 30 minutes. Preheat oven to 400°F. Bake 18–25 minutes, or until golden brown. Let cool 5 minutes; remove from pan and peel off parchment paper; cool on wire rack.

Soft Bread Dough

Generally, the softer and stickier the dough is for a yeast bread, the coarser the bread texture will be. For focaccia, you want a very coarse bread with lots of big yeast holes and a chewy texture. You can't knead this bread, so beat with an electric mixer for 3 minutes, or beat vigorously by hand for 300 strokes.

Crisp Pizza Crust

*Pizza night just got easier with this delicious, Crisp Pizza Crust
that will hold up to whatever toppings you put on it.*

INGREDIENTS | SERVES 16

1½ cups brown rice flour

½ cup potato starch

¼ cup tapioca starch

1½ teaspoons xanthan gum

1 tablespoon rapid-rise yeast

1 teaspoon salt

1 teaspoon granulated sugar

1 teaspoon Italian seasoning (optional)

½ teaspoon garlic powder (optional)

3 tablespoons olive oil

1 large egg

1¼–1½ cups warm water (start with 1¼
  cups, adding more if necessary)

Make Your Own Ready-to-Use Pizza Crusts

Make several of these crusts and freeze them, and then you can make homemade pizza in minutes. Prebake the crust for 10 minutes, and cool them completely. Wrap par-baked crusts in waxed paper and place in large freezer bags. Label, seal, and freeze the crusts for up to 6 months. To use, bake the frozen crust for another 5 minutes at 425°F, then top, and finish baking.

1. In the bowl of a stand mixer, add all the dry ingredients. Stir to combine.

2. With the mixer running, add the olive oil, egg, and 1¼ cups water, adding up to ¼ cup more water, as needed. The dough should become a nice, smooth dough, similar to a thick cake batter. Beat on medium-high speed for 3 minutes.

3. Using a rubber spatula or offset spatula dipped in water, spread the pizza crust dough out evenly on a parchment paper–lined baking sheet (two 14" round pizzas, or one large rectangle pizza).

4. Allow dough to rise for 30 minutes in a warm, draft-free place.

5. Preheat oven to 425°F.

6. Bake pizza crust in the preheated oven for 10 minutes. Remove from oven and top with your favorite sauce and toppings. Return to oven and bake until toppings are bubbling and cheese is starting to brown (another 10–15 minutes, depending on your toppings).

7. Remove from oven, let sit for 5 minutes, and then cut into slices. Carefully slide a wire cooling rack underneath the parchment paper, to allow steam to escape. If you leave the pizza (and parchment) directly on the baking sheet, steam will build up and your crust will not stay crisp.

Vanilla Scones

Thick, puffy scones are perfect for breakfast, brunch, or just as an afternoon snack. If you don't have access to vanilla beans, adding an additional teaspoon of good vanilla extract will still give a good vanilla flavor.

INGREDIENTS | SERVES 8

1¼ cups brown rice flour

¼ cup tapioca starch

4 teaspoons xanthan gum

2 teaspoons baking powder

1 teaspoon baking soda

½ teaspoon salt

¼ cup granulated sugar

1 vanilla bean, scraped

½ cup cold butter, cut into chunks

2 large eggs

½ cup sour cream or plain yogurt

1 teaspoon vanilla extract

1 egg white (for brushing)

1 tablespoon coarse sugar, for sprinkling on top (optional)

1 vanilla bean, scraped

¾ cup confectioners' sugar

1 tablespoon milk or cream

How to Scrape Out a Vanilla Bean

Inside those long, dark, dried out bean pods is a dark paste filled with tiny little vanilla seeds. To remove the seeds from the pod, simply cut the bean in half lengthwise, separate the two pieces, and use the back of a knife to scrape out the seeds from the bean. When the seeds have been scraped out, you don't have to throw the pod out. You can place the scraped-out bean into a container with granulated sugar, letting it sit for 2 weeks or more. The vanilla pod gives the sugar a beautiful vanilla flavor and aroma. This sugar can be used the same way you would use any sugar, it just has a slight vanilla flavor.

1. Preheat the oven to 425°F. Line a baking sheet with parchment paper and sprinkle with brown rice flour. Set aside.

2. Place all of the dry ingredients, plus the seeds scraped from one vanilla bean, in the bowl of a food processor. Pulse to mix the ingredients.

3. Add the cold butter, and pulse until the butter is the size of a pea. Add the eggs, sour cream, and vanilla extract. Pulse again, until the dough comes together in a ball. Spoon the dough onto your baking sheet.

4. Dust your hands with flour, then form the dough into a disk, 10" round and ¾"–1" thick. Cut into 8 even wedges, and move the wedges apart, so they are not touching.

5. Brush the tops of the scones with the egg white, and sprinkle with the coarse sugar.

6. Bake in preheated oven for 13–16 minutes, or until the tops are a nice golden brown. Remove from oven, and move scones to wire cooling rack for 15 minutes before topping with the vanilla drizzle.

7. In a small mixing bowl, stir together the seeds from one scraped vanilla bean, confectioners' sugar, and milk until the icing is smooth.

8. Place the vanilla icing into a small zipper-seal bag, and cut a small corner off the bag.

9. Place the parchment paper (that you baked the scones on) under the cooling rack that the scones are on. Drizzle the vanilla icing onto the scones.

10. Serve immediately, or store in an airtight container once the scones are completely cool. Do not stack the scones or the icing will get squished.

Banana Chocolate Chip Scones

These scones are perfect as is, or topped with some cream cheese or chocolate hazelnut spread.

INGREDIENTS | SERVES 8

1¼ cups brown rice flour

¼ cup tapioca starch

4 teaspoons xanthan gum

2 teaspoons baking powder

1 teaspoon baking soda

½ teaspoon salt

¼ cup granulated sugar

6 tablespoons cold butter, cut into chunks

1 egg yolk

1 small ripe banana, mashed (about ⅓ cup)

½ cup sour cream or plain yogurt

1 teaspoon vanilla extract

½ cup gluten-free mini chocolate chips

1 egg white (for brushing)

1. Preheat the oven to 400°F. Line a baking sheet with parchment paper and sprinkle with some brown rice flour. Set aside.

2. Place all the dry ingredients in the bowl of a food processor. Pulse to mix the ingredients.

3. Add the cold butter, and pulse until the butter is the size of a pea. Add the egg yolk, mashed banana, sour cream, vanilla extract, and mini chocolate chips. Pulse again, just until the dough comes together in a ball. Spoon the dough onto your parchment-lined baking sheet.

4. Dusting your hands with flour, quickly form the dough into a disk, about 10" round and ¾"–1" thick. Cut into 8 even wedges, and move the wedges apart, so they are not touching each other. This will allow them to bake evenly.

5. Brush the tops of the scones with the egg white.

6. Bake in preheated oven for 18–20 minutes, or until the tops are a nice golden brown. Remove from oven, and move scones to wire cooling rack for 15 minutes before serving.

7. Store in an airtight container once the scones are completely cool.

Apple Spice Bread

Applesauce and fresh apple combine in this delicious recipe to make a quick bread perfect for a snack or afterschool treat.

INGREDIENTS | SERVES 8

1 cup white rice flour

½ cup millet flour

¼ cup sorghum flour

1 teaspoon xanthan gum

¼ teaspoon salt

1 teaspoon ground cinnamon

¼ teaspoon ground nutmeg

⅛ teaspoon ground allspice

⅛ teaspoon ground cardamom

1 teaspoon baking powder

½ teaspoon baking soda

1 cup brown sugar

2 large eggs

2 tablespoons oil

1 teaspoon vanilla

½ cup unsweetened applesauce

1 cup of your favorite apple, peeled and grated

½ cup dried currants (optional)

1. Preheat oven to 350°F. Spray a 9" × 5" loaf pan with nonstick cooking spray and set aside. In a large bowl, combine flours, xanthan gum, salt, cinnamon, nutmeg, allspice, cardamom, baking powder, and baking soda; mix well.

2. In a medium bowl, combine brown sugar, eggs, oil, vanilla, applesauce, apple, and currants; mix well. Stir into dry ingredients just until mixed. Pour into prepared pan.

3. Bake 50–55 minutes, or until deep golden brown and toothpick inserted in center comes out clean. Let cool in pan for 5 minutes; remove to wire rack to cool completely.

Brown Sugar

Brown sugar can dry out quite quickly if kept in its original packaging. To make it last longer, buy a brown-sugar disc, a small pottery disc that is soaked in water. Pack the brown sugar into an airtight container and top with the disc; the brown sugar will not dry out. Make sure the cover is fastened securely and store in a cool, dark place.

Fruity Pear-Citrus Bread

Pears add moisture and flavor to this simple quick bread. You can omit the glaze if you'd like.

INGREDIENTS | SERVES 12

1½ cups white rice flour

¼ cup millet flour

¼ cup potato starch

1 teaspoon xanthan gum

½ cup granulated sugar

2 teaspoons baking powder

1 teaspoon baking soda

¼ teaspoon salt

1 teaspoon vanilla

½ cup puréed pears

1 teaspoon grated orange zest

½ cup orange juice

¼ cup oil

3 tablespoons lemon juice

1 cup powdered sugar

1. Preheat oven to 375°F. Spray a 9" × 5" loaf pan with nonstick cooking spray and set aside.

2. In a large bowl, combine flours, potato starch, xanthan gum, sugar, baking powder, baking soda, and salt; mix well.

3. In a small bowl, combine vanilla, pears, orange zest, orange juice, and oil; mix well. Add to dry ingredients and stir just until combined. Pour into prepared pan.

4. Bake 35–40 minutes, or until bread is golden brown and firm. While bread is baking, combine lemon juice and powdered sugar in a small bowl. Drizzle half of mixture over bread when it comes out of the oven.

5. Let bread cool 10 minutes in pan; remove to wire rack. Drizzle with remaining half of lemon mixture; cool completely.

Storing Quick Breads

Most quick breads, that is, breads made with baking powder or soda instead of yeast, improve in texture and flavor if allowed to stand overnight at room temperature. Cool the bread completely, then either wrap in plastic wrap or place the bread in a resealable bag. Quick breads can also be frozen for longer storage.

CHAPTER 16

Slow Cooker Recipes

Blueberry French Toast Casserole

Store-bought gluten-free bread is too expensive to waste if it becomes stale. This recipe shows you how to make a frugal but delicious breakfast or dessert using leftover or stale gluten-free bread.

INGREDIENTS | SERVES 6

7 cups gluten-free bread, cubed

1⅓ cups almond milk

5 eggs, whisked

1 tablespoon vanilla

1 tablespoon maple syrup

½ teaspoon salt

2 tablespoons butter (melted) or coconut oil

2 teaspoons cinnamon

3 tablespoons sugar

1½ cups blueberries, fresh or frozen

1. In a large bowl mix together the cubed gluten-free bread, almond milk, whisked eggs, vanilla, maple syrup, and salt.

2. Pour mixture into a greased 4-quart slow cooker.

3. Drizzle melted butter or coconut oil over the casserole. Sprinkle cinnamon and sugar evenly over the bread. Top with blueberries.

4. Cover slow cooker and vent with a wooden spoon handle or chopstick. Cook on high for 2½–3 hours or on low for 5–6 hours.

5. Remove lid and allow liquids to evaporate the last 20 minutes of cooking. Serve warm.

Breakfast Granola

Finding gluten-free granola can be a challenge in most grocery stores,
but it's super easy to make your own in the slow cooker.
Make sure to stir the ingredients about every 30 minutes to prevent uneven cooking or overbrowning.

INGREDIENTS | SERVES 10

2½ cups gluten-free rolled oats

¼ cup ground flaxseed

½ cup unsweetened shredded coconut

½ cup pumpkin seeds

½ cup walnuts, chopped

½ cup sliced almonds

1 cup dried cranberries

¾ cup brown sugar

⅓ cup coconut oil

¼ cup honey

½ teaspoon salt

1 teaspoon ground cinnamon

Change It Up

Don't like pumpkin seeds, walnuts, or dried cranberries? Use the seeds, nuts, and dried fruit that you prefer in your own granola. Use raisins, sunflower seeds, cocoa nibs, dried cranberries, or even dried bananas. The different variations are endless. You can even add chocolate chips if you'd like, but only after the granola has been cooked and cooled!

1. Mix all ingredients together and place in a greased 4-quart slow cooker.

2. Cover slow cooker and vent with a wooden spoon handle or a chopstick. Cook on high for 4 hours, or on low for 8 hours, stirring every hour or so.

3. When granola is toasty and done, pour it onto a cookie sheet that has been lined with parchment paper. Spread the granola out evenly over the entire sheet of parchment paper. Allow granola to cool and dry for several hours.

4. Once cooled, break granola up and place in an airtight container or a tightly sealed glass jar and store in pantry for up to 1 month. For longer storage keep granola in freezer for up to 6 months.

Pull-Apart Cinnamon Raisin Biscuits

Who ever thought you could make gluten-free biscuits in the slow cooker? Well, you can, and they turn out light and soft with a perfect crumb! To prevent the biscuits on the edge from browning too quickly, line the slow cooker with parchment paper.

INGREDIENTS | SERVES 9

1 cup brown rice flour
1 cup arrowroot starch
1 tablespoon baking powder
1 teaspoon xanthan gum
½ teaspoon salt
⅓ cup sugar
½ teaspoon ground cinnamon
⅓ cup vegetable shortening
2 eggs
¾ cup whole milk
½ cup raisins

Quick Vanilla Glaze

Impress your family by making a quick powdered sugar glaze for these lightly sweetened biscuits/buns. Mix together 1 cup of powdered sugar with 1½ tablespoons of water or milk and ½ teaspoon of vanilla extract. Drizzle artistically over warm buns and serve immediately.

1. In a large bowl whisk together the brown rice flour, arrowroot starch, baking powder, xanthan gum, salt, sugar, and cinnamon.

2. Cut in the vegetable shortening using a fork and knife, until it resembles small peas within the gluten-free flour mixture.

3. In a small bowl whisk together eggs and milk. Pour into the flour mixture and mix with a fork to combine, until the dough is like a very thick, sticky cake batter. Fold in the raisins.

4. Grease a 4-quart slow cooker and/or line with parchment paper.

5. Drop biscuit dough in balls about the size of a golf ball into the bottom of the greased slow cooker. The biscuits will touch each other and may fit quite snugly.

6. Cover slow cooker and vent lid with the handle of a wooden spoon or a chopstick. Cook biscuits on high for about 2–2½ hours or on low for around 4–4½ hours. Biscuits around the edge of the slow cooker will be more brown than those in the center. The biscuits should have doubled in size during cooking. The biscuits are done when a toothpick inserted in the center of the middle biscuit comes out clean.

7. Turn the slow cooker off and remove the insert to a heat-safe surface such as the stovetop or on top of potholders. Allow the biscuits to cool for several minutes before removing from slow cooker insert. They will "pull-apart" individually.

Sweet and Sour Mini Hot Dog Snackers

Sometimes it can be difficult to make sure certain brands of sandwich meats and hot dogs are gluten-free. To make it easier, instead of searching high and low for mini gluten-free hot dogs, simply use a brand of regular gluten-free hot dogs you trust and cut them into bite-sized pieces.

INGREDIENTS | SERVES 4

1 package gluten-free hot dogs, cut into bite-sized pieces

½ cup grape jelly

½ cup gluten-free barbecue sauce

2 tablespoons orange juice

½ teaspoon ground white pepper

1 tablespoon gluten-free Worcestershire sauce

½ teaspoon ground mustard

1. Place cut-up hot dogs into a greased 2.5-quart slow cooker.

2. In a bowl mix together the jelly, barbecue sauce, orange juice, pepper, Worcestershire sauce, and mustard. Pour over the hot dogs in the slow cooker.

3. Cover and cook on high for 3–4 hours or on low for 6–8 hours.

"Shake It and Bake It" Drumsticks

Remember that wonderful chicken seasoning from your childhood?
You can now make it gluten-free for crispy chicken drumsticks right in your slow cooker!

INGREDIENTS | SERVES 6

1 cup gluten-free corn tortilla chips, finely crushed

1½ tablespoons olive oil

½ teaspoon salt

½ teaspoon paprika

¼ teaspoon celery seeds

¼ teaspoon ground black pepper

¼ teaspoon garlic powder

½ teaspoon dried onion flakes

¼ teaspoon dried basil

¼ teaspoon dried parsley

¼ teaspoon dried oregano

6 chicken drumsticks

Make It and Shake It for Later

Double or triple the batch of the seasoned coating ingredients so in the future you can prepare this delicious gluten-free appetizer or light meal in a snap.

1. In a heavy-duty gallon-sized zip-top bag mix together the seasoning ingredients: crushed tortilla chips, olive oil, salt, paprika, celery seeds, pepper, garlic powder, onion flakes, basil, parsley, and oregano.

2. To prepare the slow cooker either wrap 4–5 small potatoes in foil and place them in the bottom of a greased 4-quart slow cooker, or make 4–5 foil balls about the size of a small potato and place them in the bottom of the slow cooker. (This will help the chicken to get a little bit crispy in the slow cooker instead of cooking in its juices.)

3. Place 2 drumsticks in the bag with the seasoning mix, seal it tightly, and shake the bag to coat the chicken. Place coated chicken drumsticks on top of the foil balls. Repeat with remaining drumsticks, 2 at a time.

4. Cover slow cooker and vent the lid with a chopstick to help release extra moisture. Cook on high for 4 hours or on low for 8 hours.

Lasagna with Spinach

There is no need to precook the gluten-free noodles in this recipe.

INGREDIENTS | SERVES 10

28 ounces low-fat ricotta cheese

1 cup defrosted and drained frozen cut spinach

1 egg

½ cup part-skim shredded mozzarella cheese

8 cups (about 2 jars) marinara sauce

½ pound uncooked gluten-free lasagna noodles

1. In a medium bowl, stir the ricotta, spinach, egg, and mozzarella.

2. Ladle a quarter of the marinara sauce along the bottom of a greased 6-quart slow cooker. The bottom should be thoroughly covered in sauce. Add a single layer of lasagna noodles on top of the sauce, breaking noodles if needed to fit in the sides.

3. Ladle an additional quarter of sauce over the noodles, covering all of the noodles. Top with half of the cheese mixture, pressing firmly with the back of a spoon to smooth. Add a single layer of lasagna noodles on top of the cheese, breaking noodles if needed to fit in the sides.

4. Ladle another quarter of the sauce on top of the noodles, and top with the remaining cheese. Press another layer of noodles onto the cheese and top with the remaining sauce. Take care that the noodles are entirely covered in sauce.

5. Cover and cook for 4–6 hours until cooked through.

Easy Italian Spaghetti

*It doesn't get any easier than this. Because this meal cooks so quickly,
you can put it together as soon as you get home from work.*

INGREDIENTS | SERVES 4

1 pound ground beef, browned

1 (16-ounce) jar marinara sauce

1 cup water

8 ounces gluten-free pasta, uncooked

½ cup grated Parmesan cheese

1. Add browned ground beef, marinara sauce, and water to a greased 4-quart slow cooker. Cook on high for 2 hours or on low for 4 hours.

2. Forty-five minutes prior to serving, stir dry gluten-free pasta into meat sauce. The pasta will cook in the sauce. Serve with Parmesan cheese sprinkled on top of each serving.

Retro Tuna Pasta Casserole

The popular tuna casserole can now be made gluten-free! In this recipe the pasta is cooked separately, so it doesn't become overcooked in the casserole.

INGREDIENTS | SERVES 4

2 cans water-packed white tuna, drained and flaked

1 cup heavy cream

¾ cup mayonnaise

4 hard-boiled eggs, chopped

1 cup finely diced celery

½ cup finely minced onion

1 cup frozen garden peas

¼ teaspoon ground black pepper

1½ cups crushed potato chips, divided

2 cups gluten-free pasta, cooked

1. In a large bowl combine tuna, cream, mayonnaise, eggs, celery, onion, peas, ground pepper, and ¾ cup crushed potato chips.

2. Pour tuna mixture into a greased 4-quart slow cooker. Top with remaining potato chips. Cover and cook on low for 3 hours or on high for 1½ hours.

3. To serve: place tuna casserole on top of ½ cup of pasta per person.

Biscuit-Topped Chicken Pie

Pure comfort food! This creamy chicken and vegetable pie is topped with homemade gluten-free buttermilk drop biscuits. To make the pie extra rich, drizzle a few tablespoons of melted butter over the biscuit topping right before cooking.

INGREDIENTS | SERVES 6

4 tablespoons brown rice flour

4 tablespoons butter

1 cup whole milk

1 cup gluten-free chicken broth

1 teaspoon salt

½ teaspoon ground black pepper

2 cups cooked chicken breast, cut or torn into bite-sized pieces

1 (12-ounce) can mixed vegetables, drained

1 prepared batch of dough for Fluffy Buttermilk Biscuits (see Chapter 15)

Gluten-Free Baking Mixes

Instead of homemade biscuits, you can also use your favorite gluten-free biscuit baking mix. It must be an all-purpose mix that includes xanthan gum and a leavening ingredient such as baking powder or baking soda. Use a recipe on the package that will make 8–10 gluten-free biscuits as a topping for chicken pie.

1. In a small saucepan over medium heat, whisk together flour and butter. When butter has melted, slowly stir in milk, chicken broth, salt, and pepper. Cook on medium heat for 5–10 minutes, whisking constantly until mixture is thick, with a gravy consistency.

2. Add chicken and vegetables to a greased 4-quart slow cooker. Pour creamy sauce into the slow cooker and mix with chicken and vegetables.

3. Using an ice cream scoop, drop biscuit dough over chicken, vegetables, and sauce.

4. Cover slow cooker and vent lid with a chopstick. Cook on high for 3–4 hours or on low for 6–8 hours until chicken sauce is bubbling up around the biscuits, and the biscuits are cooked through.

Chicken Alfredo Pasta

Quartered artichokes add a tangy flavor to this easy pasta casserole.

INGREDIENTS | SERVES 4

1 pound boneless skinless chicken thighs, cut into ¾-inch pieces

1 (14-ounce) can quartered artichokes, drained

1 (16-ounce) jar gluten-free Alfredo pasta sauce

1 cup water

½ cup sun-dried tomatoes, drained and chopped

8 ounces gluten-free pasta, uncooked

2 tablespoons shredded Parmesan cheese

1. In a greased 4-quart slow cooker, mix chicken, artichokes, Alfredo sauce, and water. Cover and cook on high for 3 hours or on low for 6 hours.

2. Stir tomatoes and uncooked pasta into chicken mixture 45 minutes before serving.

3. Cover lid and continue to cook until pasta is al dente. Sprinkle Parmesan cheese over individual servings.

Make Your Own Alfredo Sauce

Most Alfredo sauces are naturally gluten-free: they're usually made with butter, cheese, cream, and spices. To make your own, whisk together over medium heat: ½ cup butter, 8 ounces of light cream cheese, 1 cup whole milk or half-and-half, ⅓ cup Parmesan cheese, and 1 tablespoon of garlic powder. Allow the mixture to cool. It will thicken as it cools.

Cheesy Potato Wedges

Who doesn't like fries? Kids are especially fond of these salty, usually crispy treats.
While these potatoes don't crisp up as much as fried ones, they are definitely a salty, cheesy,
and delicious treat that's much healthier than fast food!

INGREDIENTS | SERVES 4

2 pounds red potatoes
2 teaspoons dried onions
1 teaspoon oregano
½ teaspoon garlic salt
½ teaspoon black pepper
2 tablespoons olive oil
¼ cup grated Parmesan cheese

1. Wash and scrub potatoes. Pat dry and cut into ½" wedges.

2. Place dried onions, oregano, garlic salt, and pepper in a gallon-sized zip-top bag. Add the potatoes to the bag and shake to coat the potatoes.

3. Pour the potatoes into a greased 4-quart slow cooker. Drizzle with olive oil.

4. Cover and cook on high for 4 hours or on low for 6–8 hours. Midway through the cooking process lift the lid of the slow cooker and carefully pour out any liquids that have collected on the bottom. Cover and resume cooking until potatoes are fork tender.

5. Place potatoes on a platter and sprinkle with Parmesan cheese and additional salt and pepper if needed.

Shortcut Chicken Parmesan

With a savory Italian sauce and lots of gooey mozzarella cheese, you'll never miss the breading in this recipe! Serve it with gluten-free garlic bread and steamed broccoli.

INGREDIENTS | SERVES 4

2 pounds boneless, skinless chicken breasts

1 (15-ounce) can tomato sauce

1 (4-ounce) can tomato paste

1 tablespoon Italian seasoning

½ teaspoon dried basil

½ teaspoon garlic powder

½ teaspoon salt

½ teaspoon ground pepper

2 cups shredded mozzarella

½ cup grated Parmesan cheese

1. Place chicken in the bottom of a greased 4-quart slow cooker.

2. In a large bowl mix together tomato sauce, tomato paste, Italian seasoning, basil, garlic powder, salt, and pepper. Pour sauce over chicken. Cook on high for 3–4 hours or on low for 5–6 hours.

3. An hour prior to serving sprinkle cheeses on top of the tomato sauce. Cook for 45 minutes to an hour until cheeses are melted and gooey.

Slow Cooker Yeast Bread

Did you know you can make gluten-free sandwich bread right in your slow cooker? If using the loaf pan for this bread, make sure to use the size recommended in the recipe. Otherwise, your bread can rise too high and then fall while baking.

INGREDIENTS | SERVES 12

⅓ cup arrowroot starch

⅓ cup blanched almond flour

3 tablespoons millet flour

1½ cups brown rice flour

1 teaspoon salt

1 tablespoon xanthan gum

2 teaspoons bread machine yeast (try: Saf, Red Star, or Fleischmann's)

3 tablespoons sugar

1 egg, plus 2 egg whites, room temperature

1⅓ cups whole milk, heated to 110°F

3 tablespoons olive oil

Free-Form Oval Bread

If you don't have a large 6-quart slow cooker, simply line a 2.5-quart or a 4-quart slow cooker with parchment paper. Spray it with nonstick cooking spray. Coat your hands or a large spoon with cooking spray or olive oil and shape the dough into an oval loaf. Place loaf in the middle of the parchment paper and bake. You will need to keep a close eye on the loaf as it can burn around the edges since it's closer to the heating element.

1. In a large bowl whisk together arrowroot starch, blanched almond flour, millet flour, brown rice flour, salt, xanthan gum, yeast, and sugar.

2. In a smaller bowl whisk together the egg, egg whites, milk, and oil.

3. Pour wet ingredients into whisked dry ingredients. Stir with a wooden spoon or a fork for several minutes until dough resembles a thick cake batter. First it will look like biscuit dough, but after a few minutes it will appear thick and sticky.

4. Line an 8½" × 4½" metal or glass loaf pan with parchment paper or spray with nonstick cooking spray. Pour bread dough into the pan. Using a spatula that's been dipped in water or coated with oil or nonstick cooking spray, spread the dough evenly in the pan. Continue to use the spatula to smooth out the top of the bread dough. Place the loaf pan in a 6-quart or larger oval slow cooker.

5. Cover the slow cooker and vent the lid with a chopstick or the handle of a wooden spoon. Cook on high for 3½–4 hours. The bread will rise and bake at the same time. The bread should be about double in size and the sides should be a light golden brown; the bread will not "brown" as much as it would in the oven.

6. Remove the bread from the pan and cool on a wire rack. Slice and keep in an airtight plastic bag on the counter for 2 days. Freeze any remaining bread.

Slow Cooker Yeast Rolls

This recipe proves how versatile gluten-free yeast dough can be, even in the slow cooker! You will need 2 (4-quart) slow cookers or 1 (6-quart) slow cooker for this recipe.

INGREDIENTS | SERVES 12

1 recipe gluten-free Slow Cooker Yeast Bread dough (see recipe in this chapter)

3 tablespoons olive oil or melted butter

½ teaspoon garlic powder

½ teaspoon toasted sesame seeds

½ teaspoon Italian seasoning

Drop Rolls

Instead of using cupcake liners you can simply line the slow cooker with parchment paper. Spray the parchment paper with nonstick cooking spray and drop the scoops of dough onto the parchment paper. Bake as directed.

1. Using an ice cream scoop, scoop dough into 12 balls and place each ball in a greased cupcake liner. Place the cupcake liners on the bottom of one large or two smaller slow cookers.

2. Brush rolls with melted butter and sprinkle garlic powder, sesame seeds, and/or Italian seasoning over the tops.

3. Cover and vent the lid with a chopstick or the handle of a wooden spoon. Cook on high for 1½–2½ hours until dough has almost doubled in size and the rolls are cooked through. You will need to watch the rolls at the end of the cooking period as they can get overdone on the edges since they are so close to the cooking element.

Hatteras Clam Chowder

This cozy, creamy chowder is thickened only by potatoes.
Serve it with a fresh green salad and homemade gluten-free bread.

INGREDIENTS | SERVES 4

4 slices bacon, diced

1 small onion, diced

2 medium russet potatoes, peeled and diced

1 (8-ounce) bottle clam stock

2–3 cups water

½ teaspoon salt

½ teaspoon freshly ground pepper

2 (6.5-ounce) cans minced clams (do not drain)

1. In a 2-quart or larger saucepan, sauté bacon until crispy and browned. Add onion and sauté until translucent, about 3–5 minutes. Add cooked onions and bacon to a greased 2.5-quart slow cooker.

2. Add potatoes, clam stock, and enough water to cover (2–3 cups). Add salt and pepper.

3. Cover and cook on high for 3 hours until potatoes are very tender.

4. One hour prior to serving add in the clams along with broth from the cans and cook until heated through.

Spicy Vegetarian Chili

*Have a chili party and offer diners their choice of a hearty beef chili
and this zesty and flavorful vegetarian chili.*

INGREDIENTS | SERVES 8

2 tablespoons olive oil

1½ cups chopped yellow onion

1 cup chopped red bell pepper

2 tablespoons minced garlic

2 serrano peppers, seeded and minced

1 medium zucchini, diced

2 cups frozen corn

1½ pounds portobello mushrooms
(about 5 large), stemmed, cleaned, and
cubed

2 tablespoons chili powder

1 tablespoon ground cumin

1½ teaspoons salt

¼ teaspoon cayenne pepper

2 (15-ounce) cans diced tomatoes

2 (15-ounce) cans black beans

1 (15-ounce) can tomato sauce

2 cups vegetable stock, or water

¼ cup chopped fresh cilantro leaves

1. In a large, heavy pot, heat the oil over medium-high heat. Add the onions, bell peppers, garlic, and serrano peppers, and cook, stirring, until soft, about 3 minutes.

2. Add softened vegetables to a greased 4–6-quart slow cooker. Add remaining ingredients, except for cilantro.

3. Cover and cook on high for 4–6 hours or on low for 8–10 hours. Stir in cilantro before serving.

Pick Your Own Garnishes

A fun way to serve this chili is to prepare and chill bowls of chopped avocados, sour cream, shredded cheese, crushed tortilla chips, and salsa. Allow diners to garnish their own bowls of chili when it's time to eat.

Cottage Pie with Carrots, Parsnips, and Celery

Cottage pie is similar to the more familiar shepherd's pie, but it uses beef instead of lamb.
This version uses lots of vegetables and lean meat.

INGREDIENTS | SERVES 6

1 large onion, diced

3 cloves garlic, minced

1 carrot, diced

1 parsnip, diced

1 stalk celery, diced

1 pound lean ground beef

1½ cups gluten-free beef stock

½ teaspoon hot paprika

½ teaspoon crushed rosemary

1 tablespoon gluten-free Worcestershire sauce

½ teaspoon dried savory

⅛ teaspoon salt

½ teaspoon freshly ground black pepper

1 tablespoon cornstarch and 1 tablespoon water, mixed (if necessary)

¼ cup minced fresh parsley

2¾ cups plain mashed potatoes

1. Sauté the onion, garlic, carrot, parsnip, celery, and beef in a large nonstick skillet until the ground beef is browned, about 5–6 minutes. Drain off any excess fat and discard it. Place the mixture into a greased 4-quart slow cooker.

2. Add the stock, paprika, rosemary, Worcestershire sauce, savory, salt, and pepper to the slow cooker. Cook on low for 6–8 hours. If the meat mixture still looks very thin, create a slurry by mixing together 1 tablespoon cornstarch and 1 tablespoon water. Stir this into the meat mixture.

3. In a medium bowl, mash the parsley and potatoes using a potato masher. Spread on top of the ground beef mixture in the slow cooker. Cover and cook on high for 30–60 minutes or until the potatoes are warmed through.

Save Time in the Morning

Take a few minutes the night before cooking to cut up any vegetables you need for a recipe. Place them in an airtight container or plastic bag and refrigerate until morning. Measure any dried spices and place them in a small container on the counter until needed.

Cheddar-Baked Hominy

Hominy is a wonderful, naturally gluten-free alternative to regular wheat pasta. Try it in this macaroni and cheese–inspired dish.

INGREDIENTS | SERVES 6

1½ cups whole milk

2 tablespoons cornstarch

1½ tablespoons butter

2 cups shredded Cheddar cheese, divided

1 (29-ounce) can white or yellow hominy, drained

1 egg, beaten

½ teaspoon sea salt

1 teaspoon freshly ground pepper

1 teaspoon garlic powder

¼ cup gluten-free bread crumbs or crushed tortilla chips

1. In a small bowl whisk together milk and cornstarch. Melt butter in a medium-sized saucepan and heat until sizzling. Add milk and cornstarch mixture. Whisk constantly until mixture thickens.

2. When thickened, add 1½ cups cheese. Stir together until you have a thick cheesy sauce. Add drained hominy and mix thoroughly into sauce. Add beaten egg. Stir in salt, pepper, and garlic powder.

   Pour mixture into a greased 4-quart slow cooker and sprinkle with bread crumbs or crushed tortilla chips. Cover and vent lid with a chopstick. Cook on low for 3–4 hours or on high for 2–2½ hours.

3. Thirty minutes prior to serving sprinkle remaining shredded cheese on top of casserole. Cover with lid and cook for 25–30 minutes until cheese has melted.

Rotisserie-Style Chicken

Here is a delicious alternative to buying rotisserie chicken in your grocery store. This flavorful roast chicken is incredibly easy to make in your slow cooker. For a fast weeknight meal, cook the chicken overnight in the slow cooker and serve for dinner the next day.

INGREDIENTS | SERVES 6

1 (4-pound) whole chicken
1½ teaspoons salt
2 teaspoons paprika
½ teaspoon onion powder
½ teaspoon dried thyme
½ teaspoon dried basil
½ teaspoon white pepper
½ teaspoon ground cayenne pepper
½ teaspoon black pepper
½ teaspoon garlic powder
2 tablespoons olive oil

Gravy

If you would like to make a gravy to go with the chicken, follow these directions: After removing the cooked chicken, turn slow cooker on high. Whisk ⅓ cup garbanzo bean flour or ⅓ cup brown rice flour into the cooking juices. Add salt and pepper to taste and cook for 10–15 minutes, whisking occasionally, until sauce has thickened. Spoon gravy over chicken.

1. Rinse chicken in cold water and pat dry with a paper towel.

2. In a small bowl mix together salt, paprika, onion powder, thyme, basil, white pepper, cayenne pepper, black pepper, and garlic powder.

3. Rub spice mixture over entire chicken. Rub part of the spice mixture underneath the skin, making sure to leave the skin intact.

4. Place the spice-rubbed chicken in a greased 6-quart slow cooker. Drizzle olive oil evenly over the chicken. Cook on high for 3–3½ hours or on low for 4–5 hours.

5. Remove chicken carefully from the slow cooker and place on a large plate or serving platter.

Creamy Chicken in a Mushroom and White Wine Sauce

*Many traditional slow cooker recipes call for using canned cream soups,
which often contain wheat flour as an ingredient. For a gluten-free version,
this recipe shows you how to make a simple homemade cream soup using cornstarch and milk.*

INGREDIENTS | SERVES 4

4 boneless chicken breasts, cut into chunks

3 tablespoons cornstarch

1 cup 2% milk

½ cup white wine

½ teaspoon salt

½ teaspoon ground pepper

1½ teaspoons poultry seasoning

½ teaspoon garlic powder

½ teaspoon salt-free, all-purpose seasoning

2 (4-ounce) cans sliced mushrooms, drained and rinsed

1½ cups frozen peas

2 cups cooked gluten-free pasta

1. Grease a 4-quart slow cooker with nonstick cooking spray. Place chicken into the slow cooker.

2. In a saucepan whisk together the cornstarch, milk, and white wine. Whisk in salt, pepper, poultry seasoning, garlic powder, and salt-free seasoning. Cook over medium heat whisking constantly until sauce thickens. Pour sauce over chicken.

3. Add mushrooms on top of the chicken. Cook on low for 6 hours or on high for 3 hours.

4. One hour before serving stir in the frozen garden peas.

5. Serve over pasta.

Honey-Glazed Chicken Drumsticks

It can be a challenge to eat at Chinese restaurants when you are avoiding gluten. But this Asian-inspired chicken is a great substitute for takeout! Serve with white rice, a salad, and egg drop soup.

INGREDIENTS | SERVES 4

2 pounds chicken drumsticks
1 tablespoon melted butter
¼ cup lemon juice
¾ cup honey
1 teaspoon sesame oil
3 cloves garlic, crushed
½ teaspoon ground ginger
½ teaspoon salt

1. Place chicken drumsticks in a greased 4-quart slow cooker.

2. In a glass measuring cup whisk together the melted butter, lemon juice, honey, sesame oil, garlic, ginger, and salt.

3. Pour the honey sauce over the drumsticks. Cook on high for 3–4 hours or on low for 6–8 hours.

Sesame Oil

Sesame oil is a highly flavored oil made from pressing either toasted or plain sesame seeds. It provides a unique nutty and earthy flavor to savory dishes. A little goes a long way and it's not very expensive. It can be found at most grocery stores in the Asian aisle.

Chocolate Bread Pudding

*Fat-free evaporated milk gives this bread pudding a creamy texture,
but it has several dozen fewer calories than heavy cream.*

INGREDIENTS | SERVES 10

4 cups cubed gluten-free bread, day-old
  and toasted

2⅓ cups fat-free evaporated milk

2 eggs

⅓ cup light brown sugar

¼ cup cocoa

1 teaspoon vanilla extract

1. Grease a 4-quart slow cooker with nonstick cooking spray. Add the bread cubes.

2. In a medium bowl, whisk the evaporated milk, eggs, brown sugar, cocoa, and vanilla until the sugar and cocoa are dissolved. Pour over the bread cubes.

3. Cover and cook on low for 5 hours or until the pudding no longer looks wet.

CHAPTER 17

Desserts

Cranberry Squares

Tart dried cranberries are cooked in tempting brown sugar syrup laced with just a hint of cinnamon. Leftovers, should there be any, can be covered and stored on the counter.

INGREDIENTS | SERVES 15

½ cup butter, softened
⅔ cup packed brown sugar
1¼ cups brown rice flour
½ cup potato starch
¼ cup tapioca starch
1 teaspoon xanthan gum
½ teaspoon salt
1½ cups packed brown sugar
2 tablespoons brown rice flour
½ teaspoon baking powder
¼ teaspoon salt
1 teaspoon ground cinnamon
¼ cup butter, softened
4 large eggs, beaten
2 teaspoons vanilla
3 cups dried, sweetened cranberries

1. Preheat oven to 350°F.

2. Cream ½ cup butter and ⅔ cup brown sugar together in a medium bowl. Add 1¼ cups brown rice flour, potato starch, tapioca starch, xanthan gum, and ½ teaspoon salt. Stir until well combined and crumbly. The mixture is very dry looking, but don't worry. Reserve 1 cup of the crumbs to sprinkle over the top of the squares. Press the rest of the crumbs into the bottom of a 9" × 13" baking pan. Bake the crust for 12–15 minutes, or until it is a pale golden around the edges.

3. In a medium bowl, combine 1½ cups brown sugar, 2 tablespoons brown rice flour, baking powder, ¼ teaspoon salt, and ground cinnamon. Add butter, eggs, and vanilla and stir until well blended. Stir in the dried cranberries.

4. Pour filling over the crust, top with reserved crumbles, and bake for 20–25 minutes, or until golden and bubbly around the edges but still slightly jiggly in the center. Cool completely in the pan on a wire rack. Slice into squares.

Lemon Bars

These lemon bars surpass any that you've ever had before.
The thick, tangy filling really is the best part.

INGREDIENTS | SERVES 15

1 cup unsalted butter, at room temperature

½ cup granulated sugar

1¼ cups plus 2 tablespoons brown rice flour

¼ cup plus 2 tablespoons potato starch

¼ cup tapioca starch

½ teaspoon xanthan gum

Pinch salt

7 large eggs, at room temperature

2½ cups granulated sugar

2 tablespoons grated lemon zest (approximately 4–6 lemons)

1 cup freshly squeezed lemon juice (approximately 6 lemons)

⅔ cup brown rice flour

3 tablespoons potato starch

2 tablespoons tapioca starch

Confectioners' sugar for dusting

Best Made Ahead

Lemon bars are best if you can make them one day before you are serving them. Refrigerating them will make them easier to cut. Do not sprinkle with the confectioners' sugar until you are ready to serve, as it tends to dissolve from the moisture of the lemon layer. If it does disappear before you serve it, simply sprinkle with more confectioners' sugar.

1. Preheat oven to 350°F.

2. Line a 9" × 13" baking pan with parchment paper, so the paper rises up the 13" sides. This will make removing the squares much easier, as you can lift them out once they are cooled.

3. For the crust, in the bowl of a stand mixer, cream the butter and ½ cup sugar until light and fluffy. In medium-sized bowl, combine 1¼ cups plus 2 tablespoons brown rice flour, ¼ cup plus 2 tablespoons potato starch, ¼ cup tapioca starch, xanthan gum, and salt. Slowly add to the butter/sugar mixture while the mixer is on low. Mix just until it is combined. Dump the dough into your 9" × 13" pan, and using hands dusted with rice flour, press the dough evenly over the bottom of the pan, building up ½" edge on all sides.

4. Bake in a preheated oven for 20 minutes, or until very lightly browned. Remove from oven and cool on wire rack. Do not turn the oven off yet.

5. While the crust is baking, prepare the filling. For the filling, whisk together the eggs, 2½ cups sugar, lemon zest, lemon juice, ⅔ cup brown rice flour, 3 tablespoons potato starch, and 2 tablespoons tapioca starch. Gently pour over your prebaked crust and bake for 30–35 minutes, until the filling is set. Let cool completely and refrigerate for at least 3 hours.

6. To remove from pan, cut along 9" edges, and use the parchment paper to lift the bars out to a cutting board. Using a sifter or wire sieve, dust the top of the bars with confectioners' sugar. Cut into squares, and serve.

Six-Layer Dessert

This rich, decadent dessert is always a favorite. To make it even more tempting, top it with chopped gluten-free candy bars or shaved chocolate. No one can resist.

INGREDIENTS | SERVES 15

⅔ cup brown rice flour

3 tablespoons potato starch

2 tablespoons tapioca starch

¼ teaspoon xanthan gum

2 tablespoons granulated sugar

½ cup finely chopped pecans

½ cup butter, melted

1 (8-ounce) package cream cheese, softened

1 cup confectioners' sugar

1 cup whipping cream

2 tablespoons granulated sugar

1 (3.9-ounce) package gluten-free instant chocolate pudding mix (dry)

1½ cups milk

1 (3.9-ounce) package gluten-free instant vanilla pudding mix (dry)

1½ cups milk

Finely chopped gluten-free chocolate candy or chocolate shavings (optional)

1. Preheat oven to 325°F.

2. In a small bowl, mix together brown rice flour, potato starch, tapioca starch, xanthan gum, and 2 tablespoons granulated sugar. Add chopped nuts. Stir in melted butter until all the ingredients are combined. Press mixture into a greased 9" x 13" pan.

3. Bake in preheated oven for 15 minutes. Remove and allow to cool completely.

4. Beat together the softened cream cheese and confectioners' sugar until smooth and carefully spread over cooled crust.

5. Whip cream and 2 tablespoons granulated sugar until stiff peaks form. Spread half of whipped cream over cream cheese layer.

6. In a small bowl, whisk together chocolate pudding mix and 1½ cups cold milk until smooth and just starting to set up. Carefully pour over whipped cream layer.

7. In another small bowl, whisk together vanilla pudding mix and 1½ cups cold milk until smooth and just starting to set up. Carefully pour over the chocolate pudding layer (which has had a few minutes to further set up). Top with remaining whipped cream.

8. Sprinkle the top with chopped candy or shaved chocolate, if you desire. Cover and refrigerate overnight before serving.

Blueberry Mango Crisp

The topping on this crisp can be used on any kind of fresh fruit crisp.
If you cannot tolerate gluten-free oats, you can substitute quinoa flakes for them.

INGREDIENTS | SERVES 6

1 cup granulated sugar

1 tablespoon cornstarch

1 teaspoon ground cinnamon

2 mangoes, peeled and diced to ½" pieces

4 cups blueberries

2 teaspoons vanilla

1 cup certified gluten-free oats

½ cup brown rice flour

½ cup packed brown sugar

½ teaspoon ground cinnamon

Pinch nutmeg

½ cup cold butter

Tip for Easy Cleanup

Place the 8" × 8" baking dish on a larger cookie sheet to bake. That way, if your fruit juice bubbles over while baking, it will not be in the bottom of your oven, and clean-up will be much easier.

1. Preheat oven to 350°F.

2. In a large bowl, stir together the granulated sugar, cornstarch, and 1 teaspoon cinnamon. Add the diced mango, blueberries, and vanilla. Stir to coat the fruit with the sugar mixture. Pour into an 8" × 8" baking dish and set aside.

3. To make the crisp topping, stir together the oats, brown rice flour, brown sugar, ½ teaspoon cinnamon, and pinch of nutmeg. Using a pastry cutter or two knives, cut the cold butter into the oat/flour mixture until large crumbs, about the size of a pea, remain.

4. Sprinkle the crisp topping over the top of the fruit in the baking dish, and spread to create an even layer.

5. Bake in preheated oven for 40–45 minutes, or until the fruit is hot and bubbly.

6. Remove from oven and allow to cool for at least 15 minutes before serving, as the fruit sauce is very hot straight out of the oven. This is delicious served warm with a scoop of vanilla ice cream.

Crisp Chocolate Wafers

These Crisp Chocolate Wafers can be crushed into crumbs to use as a base for a cheesecake, no-bake pie, or other dessert that calls for chocolate cookie crumbs. Or, use them to make homemade sandwich cookies or ice cream sandwiches.

INGREDIENTS | MAKES 50 (2½") COOKIES

¾ cup butter or margarine

1¼ cups granulated sugar

1 tablespoon rum or 1 teaspoon rum extract (optional)

1 large egg

½ cup brown rice flour

½ cup tapioca starch

½ cup cornstarch

1 teaspoon xanthan gum

¾ cup Dutch-processed cocoa powder

1 teaspoon baking powder

1 teaspoon baking soda

¼ teaspoon salt

1. Preheat the oven to 375°F. Tear two pieces of parchment paper the size of your baking sheets.

2. In the bowl of a stand mixer fitted with a paddle attachment, beat together the butter and granulated sugar until well combined. Add the rum (or rum extract) and egg. Beat until well mixed.

3. In a medium mixing bowl, whisk together the brown rice flour, tapioca starch, cornstarch, xanthan gum, cocoa powder, baking powder, baking soda, and salt.

4. With the mixer running on medium-low, add the dry ingredients to the sugar mixture. Mix until well combined.

5. Working with a handful of dough at a time, roll out the dough directly on one of the pieces of parchment paper that you prepared. You can sprinkle the parchment paper with a light dusting of sweet rice flour, if you wish. It will make removing the excess dough a little easier. Place plastic wrap on top of the dough to keep it from sticking to the rolling pin. Reposition the plastic wrap as necessary, and keep rolling the dough out until it is about ⅛" thick.

6. Use a round cookie cutter, about 2½" wide, to cut the cookies out of the rolled dough. Leave about 1" between cookies when cutting them out. Do not remove the cookies, though. Rather, using a rubber spatula or knife, carefully remove the excess dough *around* the cookies, leaving the cookies on the parchment paper. The excess dough that is removed can be rolled out again for the next pan of cookies.

Crisp Chocolate Wafers (continued)

Make Gluten-Free Ice Cream Sandwiches

To make these cookies into ice cream sandwiches, scoop softened ice cream onto a cookie after it has cooled. Top it with another cookie. Wrap each ice cream sandwich in plastic wrap and store in the freezer. It is best to wrap and freeze the ice cream sandwiches in advance so that the cookie has a chance to soften and the ice cream has a chance to harden before they are eaten.

7. Place the parchment paper with the cookies onto a baking sheet, and bake in preheated oven for 8 minutes.

8. While the cookies are baking, you can roll out and prepare the next batch on the other piece of parchment paper.

9. Remove cookies from oven, and allow the cookies to remain on baking pan for a few minutes before removing to wire cooling rack to cool completely.

10. Repeat this process until you have baked all the cookies, rerolling the dough that you remove from between the cookies.

11. Once cookies are completely cool, you can store them in an airtight container. These cookies also freeze wonderfully.

Soft Gingersnap Cookies

The warming aroma of this spicy cookie is enough to draw everyone into the kitchen to see what's baking. These cookies work best if you refrigerate the dough for an hour before baking your cookies.

INGREDIENTS | SERVES 48

¾ cup butter, softened
1 cup granulated sugar
1 large egg
¼ cup molasses
1 cup brown rice flour
¾ cup sorghum flour
½ cup potato starch
¼ cup tapioca starch
1 teaspoon xanthan gum
1 teaspoon baking soda
2 teaspoons ground ginger
¾ teaspoon ground cinnamon
½ teaspoon ground cloves
¼ teaspoon salt
Additional sugar for rolling the cookies in

1. Preheat oven to 350°F. Line baking sheets with parchment paper. Set aside.

2. In a stand mixer, beat the butter and sugar until light and fluffy. Add in the egg and molasses. Mix until blended.

3. In a mixing bowl, whisk together the brown rice flour, sorghum flour, potato starch, tapioca starch, xanthan gum, baking soda, ginger, cinnamon, cloves, and salt.

4. Gradually add the dry ingredients to the butter mixture, mixing until well blended.

5. Cover and refrigerate dough for 1 hour.

6. Roll the dough into ¾" balls and roll to coat in the additional granulated sugar. Place on baking sheet, 2" apart.

7. Bake in preheated oven for 10–12 minutes or until puffy and lightly browned. Remove to wire racks to cool. Store in an airtight container once completely cool.

Oatmeal Chocolate Chip Cookies

These big, soft oatmeal cookies are loaded with chocolate chips.
To change things up a bit, feel free to use chopped nuts or different flavored baking chips,
such as cinnamon or butterscotch, in place of some of the chocolate chips.

INGREDIENTS | SERVES 48

1 cup butter or margarine, softened
2 cups brown sugar, packed
2 large eggs
1 teaspoon vanilla
1½ cups brown rice flour
½ cup potato starch
¼ cup tapioca starch
½ teaspoon xanthan gum
1 teaspoon baking powder
½ teaspoon baking soda
2 cups certified gluten-free quick-cook oats
2 cups gluten-free chocolate chips

Freezing Cookies

These cookies freeze remarkably well. Just place in an airtight container and they keep in the freezer for 3–4 weeks. However, you can also freeze the dough before baking! Scoop dough onto a wax paper–lined baking sheet and place in freezer. Once cookies are completely frozen, you can place them in a resealable freezer bag. Frozen dough should be used within 4–6 weeks. To bake frozen cookies, place cookies on parchment lined baking sheets, and let the dough come to room temperature before baking as per instructions.

1. Preheat oven to 350°F.

2. Cream together the softened butter and the brown sugar.

3. Add eggs, one at a time. Mix until blended. Stir in vanilla.

4. In a large bowl, combine brown rice flour, potato starch, tapioca starch, xanthan gum, baking powder, and baking soda. Stir to blend.

5. Stir dry ingredients into butter/sugar mixture.

6. Add the rolled oats and chocolate chips, and stir to combine all ingredients.

7. Using a cookie scoop (or two tablespoons), drop cookies onto parchment lined cookie sheets. Bake cookies in preheated oven for 11–12 minutes, or until they are slightly brown around the outside, but still slightly moist in the middle.

8. Allow to cool on cookie sheet for 5 minutes before transferring to a wire rack.

9. Cool completely before storing in an airtight container.

Pumpkin Snickerdoodles

These cookies are light as air, but big on flavor.
They freeze great, and are a welcome addition to a lunchbox.

INGREDIENTS | SERVES 40

½ cup butter, softened

¾ cup granulated sugar

⅓ cup pumpkin purée (not pie filling)

1 large egg

1 teaspoon vanilla extract

1⅜ cup brown rice flour

⅜ cup potato starch

¼ cup tapioca starch

1 teaspoon xanthan gum

1 teaspoon baking powder

¼ teaspoon salt

¼ teaspoon ground cinnamon

½ cup granulated sugar

1 teaspoon pumpkin pie spice

Pumpkin Pie Spice

You can make your own pumpkin pie spice by combining 2 tablespoons ground cinnamon, 2 teaspoons each ground nutmeg and ground ginger, ½ teaspoon ground allspice, and ¼ teaspoon ground cloves. Store in an airtight container in a cool, dark place.

1. In a stand mixer, fitted with a paddle attachment, beat the butter and ¾ cup granulated sugar until light and fluffy. Add the pumpkin purée, egg, and vanilla extract, and beat until well mixed, then scrape down the bowl and mix again.

2. In a separate mixing bowl, whisk together the brown rice flour, potato starch, tapioca starch, xanthan gum, baking powder, salt, and ground cinnamon.

3. With the mixer running on low, slowly add the dry ingredients to the wet ingredients. Mix until well combined. Chill dough for 1 hour.

4. Preheat your oven to 350°F and line your baking sheets with parchment paper.

5. In a small bowl, stir together the ½ cup granulated sugar and the pumpkin pie spice.

6. Form dough into 1" balls and roll dough in the sugar/pumpkin pie spice mixture. Place cookies on prepared baking sheets, with about 2" between cookies, leaving room for the cookies to spread. Lightly press down on the tops of the cookies with the bottom of a drinking glass.

7. Bake in the preheated oven for 10–14 minutes, or until the cookies are just starting to lightly brown.

8. Allow to cool on the pan for 5 minutes, before transferring to a cooling rack. Store in an airtight container, once they are fully cooled.

White Cake

Every well-stocked recipe collection should have a recipe for a white cake.
Let this recipe for this fluffy cake be yours.

INGREDIENTS | SERVES 15

1½ cups white rice flour

½ cup millet flour

¼ cup tapioca starch

1 teaspoon xanthan gum

1½ cups granulated sugar

2 teaspoons baking powder

1 teaspoon baking soda

½ teaspoon salt

½ cup unsalted butter, softened

¾ cup milk

2 teaspoons vanilla

4 egg whites

1. Preheat oven to 350°F. Spray a 13" × 9" pan with nonstick cooking spray and set aside.

2. In a large bowl, combine rice flour, millet flour, tapioca starch, xanthan gum, sugar, baking powder, baking soda, and salt and mix well with a wire whisk.

3. In a stand mixer fitted with a paddle attachment, beat the butter until fluffy. Add the flour mixture, along with the milk and vanilla. Beat until blended, and then beat on medium speed for 2 minutes.

4. Add the unbeaten egg whites, all at once, and beat 2 minutes longer. Pour batter into prepared pan. Bake 35–40 minutes, or until cake is beginning to pull away from edges and is light golden brown. Cool completely on wire rack.

Devil's Food Cake with Mocha Buttercream

This recipe can be made into a fancy two-layer cake, or baked into cupcakes, depending on the occasion.

INGREDIENTS | SERVES 16

½ cup Dutch-processed cocoa powder

½ cup hot coffee (or water)

1 cup white rice flour

½ cup potato starch

⅓ cup cornstarch

¼ cup sorghum flour

1 teaspoon xanthan gum

2 teaspoons baking powder

1 teaspoon baking soda

¼ teaspoon salt

¾ cup unsalted butter, softened

1 cup granulated sugar

¾ cup brown sugar

3 large eggs

2 teaspoons vanilla extract

1 cup milk

1. Preheat the oven to 350°F. Line two 9" round baking pans with parchment paper.

2. In a small bowl, mix together ½ cup cocoa powder and hot coffee. Let it sit for a few minutes while you prepare the other ingredients.

3. Sift together the white rice flour, potato starch, cornstarch, sorghum flour, xanthan gum, baking powder, baking soda, and salt. Set aside.

4. In the bowl of a stand mixer, beat the butter, granulated sugar, and brown sugar until light and fluffy, scraping down the bowl when necessary. Add in the eggs, one at a time, and 2 teaspoons vanilla extract. Mix until well blended.

5. Add the milk to the cocoa/coffee mixture.

6. With the stand mixer running on low, add half of the sifted dry ingredients to the mixer. Mix until nearly all blended. Add the cocoa mixture, and when that is incorporated, add the rest of the dry ingredients. Once it is all incorporated, divide the batter between the two prepared pans. Place on middle rack in preheated oven and bake for 35–40 minutes, or until a toothpick inserted into the middle of the cake comes out clean.

7. Remove cakes from oven and allow to sit for 5 minutes before running a knife around the outside of the cake, and inverting the cake onto a wire cooling rack. Cool completely before frosting.

Devil's Food Cake with Mocha Buttercream (continued)

Frosting

1 cup unsalted butter, softened

1 cup Dutch-processed cocoa powder

1 teaspoon vanilla extract

½ teaspoon instant espresso powder

4 cups sifted confectioners' sugar

4–6 tablespoons water

8. To make the frosting: with a hand mixer, beat together 1 cup butter, 1 cup cocoa powder, 1 teaspoon vanilla, espresso powder, and confectioners' sugar. Slowly add enough water to reach desired consistency. You want the frosting to be stiff enough to hold its shape, but soft enough to easily spread over the cake.

9. Use an offset spatula to frost the cake as desired.

Moist Banana Cake

This moist cake stays fresh for days on the counter. Although it doesn't require a frosting to be enjoyed, it is also tasty topped with sweetened whipped cream, or chocolate frosting.

INGREDIENTS | SERVES 15

½ cup brown rice flour

1 cup sorghum flour

¾ cup gluten-free oat flour

¼ cup tapioca starch

1 teaspoon xanthan gum

2 teaspoons baking soda

1 teaspoon baking powder

1 teaspoon espresso powder (optional)

½ teaspoon ground cinnamon

½ teaspoon salt

½ cup unsalted butter, softened

1 cup granulated sugar

¾ cup brown sugar

3 large eggs

1 teaspoon vanilla extract

3 large overripe bananas, mashed (about 2 cups total)

⅔ cup sour cream

½ cup chopped walnuts (omit for nut-free cake)

No Oats?

No problem. If you cannot find or tolerate oat flour, feel free to substitute millet flour for it.

1. Preheat the oven to 350°F, and lightly grease one 9" × 13" pan. Set aside.

2. In a large mixing bowl, whisk together the brown rice flour, sorghum flour, oat flour, tapioca starch, xanthan gum, baking soda, baking powder, espresso powder, ground cinnamon, and salt. Set aside.

3. In a separate large mixing bowl, or the bowl of a stand mixer, beat the softened butter with the granulated and brown sugar until light and fluffy.

4. In another bowl, stir to combine the eggs, vanilla, mashed bananas, and sour cream.

5. Pour the banana mixture into the butter/sugar mixture, and beat until well blended.

6. With the mixer running on medium-low speed, add the dry ingredients to the wet ingredients. Stir to combine. Add the walnuts and stir again to incorporate them.

7. Pour cake batter into prepared pan, leveling the top with a rubber spatula. Bake in preheated oven for 45–50 minutes, or until a toothpick inserted into the middle comes out clean. The cake will also release from the edge of the pan, and the top may begin to crack slightly.

8. Remove from oven and cool completely before serving.

Crustless Pumpkin Pie

*This pie has the same fantastic flavor as traditional pumpkin pie,
only it is much easier to make since it does not have a crust.*

INGREDIENTS | SERVES 8

1 (15-ounce) can pumpkin purée (not pie filling)
½ cup packed brown sugar
½ cup granulated sugar
⅛ teaspoon ground cloves
½ tablespoon ground cinnamon
1 teaspoon ground ginger
½ teaspoon salt
2 teaspoons baking powder
½ cup sorghum flour
2 tablespoons tapioca starch
2 teaspoons vanilla
2 tablespoons olive oil
2 large eggs, beaten
½ cup evaporated milk
½ cup heavy cream
Whipped cream, for topping

1. Preheat oven to 350°F.

2. Grease a 9½" pie plate with oil.

3. Combine all ingredients and mix until well combined.

4. Pour into prepared pie plate, and bake in preheated oven for 60–70 minutes. The pie is done when a knife inserted into the middle comes out clean.

5. Cool completely before serving. Serve with a dollop of whipped cream.

The Skinny on Crustless Pies

Go ahead and have that scoop of whipped cream with your pie without feeling too guilty. By removing the crust from this pie, you save nearly 1,000 calories per pie, or 125 calories per slice.

Neapolitan Cupcakes with Strawberry-Swirl Buttercream

Which is your favorite? Chocolate? Vanilla? Strawberry?
Now you don't have to pick just one—you can enjoy all three flavors in these delectable cupcakes.

INGREDIENTS | SERVES 12

⅓ cup brown rice flour

⅓ cup tapioca starch

⅓ cup sorghum flour

½ teaspoon xanthan gum

¾ cup granulated sugar

1½ teaspoons baking powder

½ teaspoon baking soda

¼ teaspoon salt

¾ cup buttermilk

¼ cup oil

2 large eggs

2 tablespoons cocoa powder

1 teaspoon vanilla extract

1 teaspoon strawberry extract plus 5 drops red food coloring

1. Preheat oven to 350°F. Line 12 muffin cups with paper liners. Set aside.

2. In a large bowl, whisk together the brown rice flour, tapioca starch, sorghum flour, xanthan gum, granulated sugar, baking powder, baking soda, and ¼ teaspoon salt.

3. In a smaller bowl, whisk together the buttermilk, oil, and eggs. Pour into the dry ingredients, and stir just until mixed. Divide the batter between three medium bowls.

4. To the batter in the first bowl, stir in the cocoa powder.

5. To the batter in the second bowl, stir in 1 teaspoon vanilla extract.

6. To the batter in the third bowl, stir in 1 teaspoon strawberry extract plus 5 drops of red coloring.

7. Scoop batter into prepared muffin cups, layering each flavor of batter. You will need about 1½ tablespoons of each flavor batter to fill the baking pans evenly.

8. Bake in preheated oven for 18–20 minutes, or until a toothpick inserted into the middle of the cupcake comes out clean. Remove from oven and allow to cool for 5 minutes before removing to wire cooling rack. Cool completely before frosting.

9. To make the buttercream, beat together the confectioners' sugar, butter, heavy cream, and a pinch of salt until smooth and fluffy (3–5 minutes with a stand mixer). Divide buttercream between two bowls.

Neapolitan Cupcakes with Strawberry-Swirl Buttercream (continued)

Frosting

3 cups confectioners' sugar, sifted

¾ cup unsalted butter, softened

3 tablespoons heavy cream

Pinch salt

1 teaspoon vanilla extract

½ teaspoon strawberry extract

10. To one bowl, incorporate 1 teaspoon of vanilla extract.

11. To the second bowl, incorporate ½ teaspoon strawberry extract.

12. Place the buttercream in a piping bag fitted with a large star tip. By placing the vanilla buttercream on one side of the piping bag, and the strawberry on the other, the two will mix in a beautiful swirl pattern when you are piping it onto the cupcakes.

13. Store frosted cupcakes in an airtight container on the counter for up to 3 days.

Chocolate Raspberry Cupcakes with Fluffy Raspberry Frosting

These cupcakes are lighter than air but they are heavy on the chocolate flavor with a hint of raspberry as well. The frosting is made pink with raspberry purée, but also gets a great raspberry flavor from some raspberry extract.

INGREDIENTS | SERVES 26

1½ cups granulated sugar
½ cup sorghum flour
½ cup brown rice flour
½ cup potato starch
¾ cup unsweetened cocoa powder
1 teaspoon xanthan gum
2 teaspoons baking soda
2 teaspoons baking powder
½ teaspoon salt
1 cup milk
2 eggs
½ cup oil
2 teaspoons raspberry extract
1 cup boiling water

No Seeds, Please

To make the frosting free from raspberry seeds, push the mashed raspberries through a mesh strainer with the back of a spoon. This will leave you with seedless raspberry purée.

1. Preheat oven to 350°F. Line muffin tins with paper liners.

2. In a large bowl, whisk together the granulated sugar, sorghum flour, brown rice flour, potato starch, cocoa powder, xanthan gum, baking soda, baking powder, and ½ teaspoon salt until evenly blended.

3. In another small bowl, whisk together the milk, eggs, oil, and 2 teaspoons raspberry extract. Pour the wet ingredients into the dry ingredients, and beat for 1 minute.

4. Add the boiling water, and using a wooden spoon, stir until it is completely mixed into the batter. The batter will be thin.

5. Fill the muffin tins with the batter until ⅔ full. Bake on the center rack of your preheated oven for about 20–22 minutes. Be sure to test if the cupcakes are completely baked by inserting a toothpick into the middle of the cupcake. If the toothpick comes out clean, the cupcakes are done. If there is still batter on the toothpick, bake for another 2 minutes and test again.

6. Remove from oven and let sit for 5 minutes before removing cupcakes to wire rack to cool completely. Do not frost cupcakes until they have cooled completely.

7. To make the frosting: in a stand mixer, fitted with a paddle attachment, beat the butter until light colored.

Chocolate Raspberry Cupcakes with Fluffy Raspberry Frosting (continued)

Frosting

1 cup unsalted butter, softened
½ teaspoon salt
4 tablespoons mashed raspberries
2 teaspoons raspberry extract
4 cups confectioners' sugar
1–2 tablespoons heavy cream or milk
26 fresh, plump raspberries (optional)

8. Add ½ teaspoon salt, raspberry purée, and 2 teaspoons raspberry extract. Beat until it is completely mixed.

9. Add the confectioners' sugar and run the mixer until it all comes together. Scrape down the sides and mix again. Add the milk, 1 tablespoon at a time, until you get the frosting the consistency that you want.

10. You can either spread the frosting on with a knife, or pipe it on with a piping bag with a large tip. Top each cupcake with a fresh raspberry (optional). Store the cupcakes in an airtight container. They are best if they are eaten in the first 2 days.

Pumpkin Cheesecake

This dessert is the perfect combination of cheesecake and pumpkin pie.
This is the perfect dessert to enjoy during fall celebrations.

INGREDIENTS | SERVES 9

¾ cup crushed Cinnamon Chex or gluten-free graham cracker crumbs

½ cup ground pecans

2 tablespoons granulated sugar

2 tablespoons brown sugar

¼ cup butter, melted

¾ cup granulated sugar

¾ cup pumpkin purée (not pie filling)

3 egg yolks

1½ teaspoons ground cinnamon

½ teaspoon ground nutmeg

½ teaspoon ground ginger

¼ teaspoon salt

3 (8-ounce) packages cream cheese

⅜ cup granulated sugar

1 large egg

1 egg yolk

2 tablespoons whipping cream

1 tablespoon cornstarch

1 teaspoon vanilla extract

Optional: Whole pecans and a jar of dulce de leche for toppings

Keeping Things Clean

To keep your oven clean when baking anything in a springform pan, place the pan on a foil-lined baking sheet. This way, if the pan does not seal properly and some of the batter leaks out, it will not be into the bottom of your oven.

1. Preheat oven to 350°F.

2. Combine the Cinnamon Chex crumbs, ground pecans, 2 tablespoons granulated sugar, 2 tablespoons brown sugar, and the melted butter and mix well. Firmly press into one 9" springform pan.

3. Combine ¾ cup granulated sugar, pumpkin purée, 3 egg yolks, spices, and salt in a medium bowl. Mix well and set aside.

4. Beat the cream cheese with an electric mixer until light and fluffy; gradually add ⅜ cup granulated sugar and mix well. Add the whole egg, remaining egg yolk, and the whipping cream, beating well. Add cornstarch and vanilla extract, and beat batter until smooth. Add pumpkin purée mixture and mix well. Pour batter into prepared pan.

5. Bake in preheated oven for 50–55 minutes. Do not overbake. The center may be soft but it will firm up when chilled. At this point, turn the oven off, and open the oven door, but leave the cake in the oven for the next hour. This will help prevent the top from cracking.

6. Cover and refrigerate until ready to serve. Remove the springform pan and decorate the top with dulce de leche and whole pecans a few hours before serving, then place in the fridge until ready to serve.

Baked Chocolate Doughnuts

One of the things you might miss most when on a gluten-free diet is doughnuts. These quick doughnuts are baked, making them a (slightly) healthier option.

INGREDIENTS | SERVES 6

½ cup brown rice flour

¼ cup sorghum flour

2 tablespoons potato starch

1 tablespoon tapioca starch

½ teaspoon xanthan gum

2 tablespoons dry gluten-free instant chocolate pudding mix (or dry milk powder)

3 tablespoons cocoa powder

½ cup granulated sugar

1 teaspoon baking powder

¼ teaspoon salt

2 large eggs

¼ cup oil

¼ cup milk

½ teaspoon apple cider vinegar

Frosting

1 cup confectioners' sugar

2 tablespoons cocoa powder

2 tablespoons butter, softened

1–2 tablespoons milk

1. Preheat your oven to 375°F. Lightly grease a doughnut pan.

2. In a large bowl, whisk together all the dry ingredients.

3. In a smaller bowl, whisk together all the wet ingredients.

4. Pour the wet ingredients into the dry ingredients and stir until fully combined.

5. Spoon mixture into prepared doughnut pan. Bake in preheated oven for 10–12 minutes, or until a toothpick inserted into the thickest part of the doughnut comes out clean.

6. Let doughnuts sit for 5 minutes before turning them out onto a cooling rack. Allow to cool completely before frosting.

7. For the frosting: stir together the confectioners' sugar, 2 tablespoons cocoa powder, butter, and enough milk to make the glaze the consistency you want. Dip your cooled doughnuts into the glaze, and top with sprinkles, chopped nuts, or shredded coconut, if you prefer.

Ultimate Monkey Bread

*While this sweet, sticky bread is perfect for a fabulous dessert,
many people also serve it on special occasions, like Christmas morning.*

INGREDIENTS | SERVES 10

½ cup chopped pecans (optional)
1¾ cups brown rice flour
½ cup potato starch
¾ cup plus 1 tablespoon tapioca starch
1 tablespoon rapid rise yeast
3 tablespoons granulated sugar
½ teaspoon salt
1 tablespoon xanthan gum
¼ cup gluten-free instant vanilla
  pudding mix (dry)
1 teaspoon baking powder
¼ cup butter
½ cup water
¾ cup milk
1 large egg, room temperature
1 teaspoon apple cider vinegar
2 tablespoons oil
1 teaspoon vanilla extract
½ cup rehydrated raisins (optional)
½ cup granulated sugar
1–2 teaspoons ground cinnamon
½ cup butter
1 cup brown sugar
2 tablespoons maple syrup
Pinch salt
½ teaspoon vanilla extract
2 tablespoons heavy cream

1. Place chopped pecans into the bottom of a bundt cake or tube pan. Set aside. Do not use a pan with a removable bottom, as the syrup would run through and make a huge mess.

2. In the bowl of your stand mixer, whisk together the next nine ingredients until combined. Set aside.

3. Put water and ¼ cup butter in a glass measuring cup and microwave just until the butter has melted. Remove from microwave and stir. Add milk, stir. Add egg, apple cider vinegar, oil, and 1 teaspoon vanilla extract and whisk to combine.

4. With the stand mixer running (using the paddle attachment), pour the wet ingredients into the dry ingredients. Scrape down the bowl if you have to. Add the raisins if using.

5. Allow to mix on medium speed for 3 minutes.

6. In a shallow bowl, stir together the ½ cup granulated sugar and ground cinnamon. Form the dough into ¾" balls and roll them to coat them fully in the cinnamon/sugar mixture.

7. Place sugar coated dough into the bundt pan, on top of the pecans. Be sure to not tightly pack the dough into the pan; allow gaps between the dough. Repeat until all the dough has been formed, rolled in the cinnamon/sugar mixture, and placed in the pan. If you have any cinnamon/sugar mixture left, sprinkle it over the top of the dough in the pan.

Ultimate Monkey Bread (continued)

Make It Ahead of Time, and Freeze It for Later

You can form the dough, get it all prepped and in the baking pan, wrap it up in plastic wrap (a few layers is best), and put it straight in the freezer. Remove your baking pan from the freezer and place it in the fridge the night before you want to serve it. This allows the dough to defrost, but not begin rising too much yet. When you are ready to bake it, place the baking pan in a warm, draft-free place and allow it to rise for 30–40 minutes, or until the dough has nearly doubled in size. Baking directions are the same as if you were to bake it immediately. Do not freeze it for longer than 1 week.

8. In a small saucepan over low heat, melt ½ cup butter. Stir in the brown sugar, maple syrup, salt, and ½ teaspoon vanilla. Stir until the sugar is dissolved. Stir in the heavy cream. Pour mixture over the top of the dough.

9. If you want to freeze the dough, now would be the time to wrap the pan in two layers of plastic wrap and place in the freezer.

10. To bake immediately, allow the dough to rise for 20–30 minutes in a warm, draft-free place. Bake in preheated 350°F oven for 30–35 minutes. When you remove the Monkey Bread from the oven, allow it to sit in the baking pan for 5 minutes before turning it out onto a serving dish or plate. To do this, place the plate upside down on top of the baking pan, and (while wearing oven mitts, just in case) quickly turn the plate and baking pan upside down. Your Monkey Bread should release from the pan without a problem. If there are still pecans and syrup in the baking pan, use a spoon and spoon the mixture over the top of the Monkey Bread. Wait 10–15 minutes before serving. This not only allows the syrup to cool off a bit, but also allows the texture of the bread to improve.

Cream Puffs (Choux Paste)

This dough, called choux paste, can be used to make both cream puffs and éclairs. To make éclairs, pipe the dough into 4" logs, about 1½" wide, and bake according to these directions.

INGREDIENTS | SERVES 12

⅔ cup white rice flour

⅓ cup sweet rice flour

½ teaspoon xanthan gum

Pinch salt

1 teaspoon baking powder

1 cup water

½ cup unsalted butter

4 large eggs, room temperature

1. Preheat the oven to 400°F. Line a baking sheet with parchment paper, and set aside.

2. In a mixing bowl, whisk together the white rice flour, sweet rice flour, xanthan gum, salt, and baking powder. Set aside.

3. In a medium saucepan, bring the water and butter to a boil. Once they have reached a boil, pour all of the dry ingredients in at once, and stir with a wooden spoon until the dry ingredients are completely incorporated, and the mixture looks similar to play dough.

4. Place hot dough into a large mixing bowl or bowl of a stand mixer fitted with a paddle attachment. Beat on medium-high speed for a minute or two to cool the dough down a bit. With the mixer on medium speed, add eggs, one at a time. Beat dough until the egg is completely incorporated before adding the next one. Repeat until all 4 eggs have been added.

5. Mix on medium-high speed for 1 minute, until the dough is smooth.

6. Spoon the dough (about ¼ cup per cream puff) onto prepared baking sheet, leaving about 2" between cream puffs.

Cream Puffs (Choux Paste) continued

How to Freeze Choux Paste

You can freeze the choux paste to bake into Cream Puffs or éclairs at a later time. While the dough is still warm, form them onto a wax paper lined baking sheet and place in the freezer. Once they are frozen, store in a resealable freezer bag. To bake, place frozen dough onto parchment-lined baking sheet, and let come to room temperature before baking (about 15 minutes). Bake the same way you would if you were baking immediately.

7. Bake in preheated oven for 30 minutes. Turn off the oven, open the door, and pierce each cream puff with a sharp knife. This will help any steam trapped inside them to escape, giving a nice crisp cream puff. Leave the cream puffs in the oven, with the door open a few inches, until the oven has cooled completely.

8. Once cream puffs have completely cooled, fill them with a sweet or savory filling. They are best served the same day, but can be stored in an airtight container. To crisp unfilled cream puffs again, place in a 400°F oven for 10 minutes.

Piña Colada Parfait

A rum-infused pineapple curd is layered with a thin cream cheese layer, and topped with coconut-flavored whipped cream, and toasted coconut flakes.

INGREDIENTS | SERVES 6

½ cup granulated sugar

1 tablespoon cornstarch

2 large eggs, beaten

½ cup rum (or more pineapple juice)

1 (19-ounce) can crushed pineapple, with juice

½ cup unsalted butter, cut into pieces

¼ cup large flaked coconut

1½ cups whipping cream

½ cup confectioners' sugar

½ teaspoon coconut extract

4 ounces cream cheese, softened

1. In a large saucepan, whisk together the granulated sugar and cornstarch. Whisk in the eggs, rum, and crushed pineapple with juice.

2. Stirring constantly with a rubber spatula or wooden spoon, heat the mixture over medium heat until it thickens, about 10 minutes. Remove from heat and stir in a few of the pieces of butter at a time, stirring until they have melted before adding more butter. Repeat until all of the butter has been melted into the curd.

3. Scrape pineapple mixture into a bowl and place plastic wrap directly over the top of the curd. This will keep a skin from forming on the curd. Place in refrigerator and cool completely.

4. To toast the coconut, place the coconut in a frying pan over medium heat. Stir and keep an eye on it until the coconut begins to brown. Remove to a plate before it darkens too much. Allow to cool.

5. In a deep bowl, beat the whipping cream, confectioners' sugar, and coconut extract with an electric mixer until stiff peaks form.

6. In another small bowl, beat the cream cheese until soft and smooth. Stir in about 1 cup of the whipped cream mixture.

7. Line up 6 serving glasses, approximately 5–6 ounces each. Carefully spoon the pineapple curd into each glass, trying to keep the sides of the glasses clean.

Piña Colada Parfait (continued)

Using Pineapple Juice

When buying canned fruit, buy varieties that are canned in natural juices instead of corn syrup. The leftover juice can be saved in the refrigerator to use later as juice to drink, or even as a natural sweetener for a glass of iced tea or a bowl of warm oatmeal.

8. The cream cheese mixture is the next layer. To get this layer into the glasses easily, place the mixture into a plastic bag and snip the corner off it. You can then pipe it in without getting the sides of the glass dirty.

9. Divide the remaining curd between the 6 glasses.

10. Carefully spoon the coconut whipped cream (or use a piping bag fitted with a large star tip) on top of the parfaits. Sprinkle each dessert with the toasted coconut.

11. Pineapple curd can be made up to 1 day in advance. The parfaits can be assembled up to 6 hours in advance (more if you don't put the whipped cream on until serving).

Blackberry-Yogurt Pops

*These ice pops are attractive and nutritious.
Blackberries are an excellent source of fiber, vitamin C, vitamin K, and folic acid.*

INGREDIENTS | SERVES 6

2 cups plain yogurt

½ cup sugar

½ cup puréed blackberries

Crack the Ice Pop Code

The secret to a good ice pop is simple: sugar. Sugar lowers the freezing point of the pop so it stays soft and smooth, not brittle like an ice cube. So resist the urge to fully eliminate sugar from ice pop recipes that call for it.

1. In a medium bowl, whisk together the yogurt and sugar until the sugar dissolves.

2. Divide half of the yogurt mixture between 6 ice pop molds. Evenly divide all of the blackberry purée between the six ice pop molds. Top with remaining yogurt mixture.

3. Insert pop sticks and freeze until solid.

CHAPTER 18

Arts and Crafts Recipes

Play Dough

Some kids can't resist eating a little bit of play dough when they're making their creations. That is one of the reasons it is important that children on a gluten-free diet use gluten-free Play Dough.

INGREDIENTS | MAKES 1½ CUPS

½ cup white rice flour

½ cup cornstarch

¼ cup salt

2 teaspoons cream of tartar

1 cup water

1 tablespoon vegetable oil

Liquid or gel food color, or 1 package dry Kool-Aid powder

½ teaspoon chunky glitter, your choice of color (optional)

Is Play-Doh Gluten-Free?

The original Play-Doh was first demonstrated and sold in 1956. According to Hasbro, who now owns the rights to Play-Doh, the formula for the original Play-Doh still remains a secret. What we do know, however, is that Play-Doh does contain wheat, making it an unsafe toy for children on a gluten-free diet.

1. In a mixing bowl, whisk together the white rice flour, cornstarch, salt, and cream of tartar. Set aside.

2. Bring the water to a boil in a large saucepan (at least 4-quart). Add the oil.

3. Stir the dry ingredients into the boiling water along with either the food coloring or Kool-Aid powder. Add the glitter, if using. Continue stirring over medium-low heat until the dough starts to appear dry.

4. Turn dough out onto a sheet of waxed paper, and continue kneading it until it is completely cool. It will be very sticky at first, but becomes less sticky as it cools.

5. Store in an airtight bag in the refrigerator and bring to room temperature before playing with it.

Sidewalk Paint

Keep the kids busy with this fun Sidewalk Paint.
No need to worry—it washes off the sidewalk with the next rain.

INGREDIENTS | MAKES ¼ CUP

4 tablespoons cornstarch

4–5 tablespoons water

5–10 drops of liquid food coloring

1. Stir together the cornstarch and 4 tablespoons water until mixture is smooth, adding another tablespoon of water if necessary. Stir in enough food coloring to make an intense color.

2. Using large paint brushes, brush the paint onto the sidewalk. As the paint dries, the color gets brighter. The paint washes away with water or the next rainfall.

Bubbles Bubbles

Whether you are young or not-so-young, making bubbles is always fun.

2 cups water

½ cup Dawn original blue dishwashing liquid (for some reason, this brand works best)

3 tablespoons light corn syrup

Bubble wands, any size or shape

1. Mix the water, dishwashing soap, and corn syrup together in an airtight container with a tight cover.

2. Once the solution is mixed well, skim the small bubbles off the top of the solution. You can either use it straight out of the container or put the solution into a shallow bowl so more people can reach it at once.

Get Creative

If you don't have an old wand left over from other jars of bubbles, you can make your own out of a wire hanger or a plastic strawberry basket. Experiment with different sizes and shapes, and see what happens!

Edible Finger Paint

This finger paint is not only great for kids avoiding gluten, but it is something everyone can enjoy. Just remember that even though this paint is edible, a lot of different hands have been in this paint, so you should limit the amount that goes into a child's mouth.

INGREDIENTS | MAKES 2 CUPS OF PAINT

1 (3.9-ounce) package gluten-free instant vanilla pudding mix

2 cups cold water

Food coloring

Make Sure It Is Safe

Not all instant pudding mixes are gluten-free, so be sure to read the ingredient list when making your purchase.

1. In a large bowl, use a whisk to combine the pudding mix with the cold water.

2. Pour the mixture into a muffin tin or several small bowls.

3. Stir several drops of food coloring into each muffin cup or bowl to make different colors.

4. Refrigerate for 10–15 minutes before painting.

Papier Mâché

Working with wheat-based papier mâché increases the chances of gluten contamination. Use this recipe to make masks or piñatas.

INGREDIENTS | MAKES 4 CUPS

½ cup cornstarch

4 cups cold water

Papier Mâché Helmets?

Papier mâché was first made in China, the inventors of paper itself. They did not use it for crafting, however. They used it to make helmets! Helmets made from papier mâché, coated in a number of layers of lacquer to give them strength, have been dated back as far as A.D. 200.

1. In a medium-sized saucepan, whisk together the cornstarch and cold water.

2. Bring the mixture to a boil over a medium-high heat, whisking constantly.

3. Once the mixture has boiled for 2 minutes, remove from heat and allow to cool until the mixture is warm, stirring occasionally. Use the mixture while it is still warm, since it thickens when cooled. Cleanup is easy with some soap and warm water.

Gluten-Free Ingredient Resources

Amazon.com

A variety of gluten-free products and ingredients can be purchased from Amazon.com.

www.amazon.com

Arrowhead Mills

Arrowhead Mills offers a wide variety of baking mixes, flours, beans, grains, and nut butters.

www.arrowheadmills.com/category/gluten-free

Only Oats by Avena Foods

Only Oats is a Canadian supplier of certified gluten-free oats, oat flour, and various baking mixes.

www.avenafoods.com

Betty Crocker

Betty Crocker now has a line of gluten-free products. Included are cake, brownie, and cookie mixes, as well as gluten-free Bisquick. These products can be found in many neighborhood grocery stores.

www.bettycrocker.com/products

Bob's Red Mill

Bob's Red Mill carries a variety of gluten-free flours, oats, baking mixes, and other ingredients.

www.bobsredmill.com

Premier Japan

Premier Japan produces gluten-free Asian sauces, such as soy sauce, hoisin sauce, and oyster sauce.

www.edwardandsons.com

GF Harvest

GF Harvest sells a variety of certified gluten-free oat products, including flour, rolled oat, groats, and granola. Products are also available to purchase in bulk.

www.glutenfreeoats.com

Glutino

Glutino offers a variety of gluten-free baking mixes, breads, frozen meals, and snacks.

www.glutino.com

King Arthur Flour

Whether you are looking for gluten-free mixes for bread, pancakes, or cake, King Arthur Flour carries them all. Available both in-store and online.

www.kingarthurflour.com/glutenfree

Kinnikinnick Foods

Although a lot of Kinnikinnick Foods products are available in stores, you can save a few dollars by ordering online. Kinnikinnick Foods carries baking mixes, breads, cookies, and snacks that are free from gluten, soy, eggs, and sesame seeds.

www.kinnikinnick.com

Namaste Foods

Namaste Foods carries a variety of baking and cooking mixes, ranging from cakes and cookies to pasta salad and macaroni and dairy-free "cheese." All of their mixes are free from wheat, gluten, corn, soy, potato, dairy, casein, tree nuts, and peanuts.

www.namastefoods.com

Pamela's Products

Pamela's Products not only has gluten-free baking mixes, but they also produce gluten-free cookies, cakes, and bars.

www.pamelasproducts.com

Tinkyáda Rice Pasta

Tinkyáda Rice Pasta produces a wide variety of rice pastas. Very often they are available in your own grocery store.

www.tinkyada.com

Resources for Gluten-Free Dining Out

Celiac Restaurant Guide

Search menus online by restaurant or location, or even find restaurants that are 100 percent gluten-free.

www.celiacrestaurantguide.com

Find Me Gluten Free

An app for your mobile device that helps you find gluten-free-friendly businesses; includes customer reviews and photos.

www.findmeglutenfree.com

Gluten Free Registry

Find gluten-free restaurants, cafés, and bakeries all in a matter of minutes. You can search directly from the website, or download the app for your mobile device.

www.glutenfreeregistry.com

Triumph Dining

You can purchase printed gluten-free restaurant and grocery guides to help you find gluten-free items quickly. They also sell dining cards that are designed to help inform the chef and wait-staff of your dietary needs.

www.triumphdining.com

Support for Those Living Gluten-Free

Canadian Celiac Association

Find local support groups through the Canadian Celiac Association, as well as updated news regarding diagnosis and testing.

www.celiac.ca

Celiac.com

Founded by Scott Adams in 1995, it's one of the oldest online resources for all information gluten-free, including the *Journal of Gluten Sensitivity*, an online gluten-free mall, and a host of gluten-free forums.

www.celiac.com

Celiac Disease Foundation

A very active gluten-free and celiac disease–awareness organization that has been in operation since 1990.

www.celiac.org

The Celiac Scene

When traveling through Canada, check The Celiac Scene for a list of gluten-free restaurants and retailers.

www.theceliacscene.com

Celiac Sprue Association (CSA)

A great resource for finding local gluten-free support groups, along with basic information on starting the gluten-free diet.

www.csaceliacs.info

Gluten Intolerance Group (GIG)

Another resource for finding local gluten-free support groups, as well as information on safe foods that are certified gluten-free by GIG programs.

www.gluten.net

National Foundation for Celiac Awareness

A nonprofit organization that supports raising awareness for celiac disease and gluten intolerance.

www.celiaccentral.org

Raising Our Celiac Kids (R.O.C.K.)

Find support groups specifically designed for kids and their families.

www.celiac.com/articles/563/1/ROCK-Raising-Our-Celiac-Kids---National-Celiac-Disease-Support-Group/Page1.html

The University of Chicago Celiac Disease Center

Striving to cure celiac disease by 2026, the University of Chicago Celiac Disease Center is a great place for doctors and patients to find information on the latest in celiac disease research.

www.cureceliacdisease.org

Standard U.S./Metric Measurement Conversions

VOLUME CONVERSIONS

U.S. Volume Measure	Metric Equivalent
⅛ teaspoon	0.5 milliliter
¼ teaspoon	1 milliliter
½ teaspoon	2 milliliters
1 teaspoon	5 milliliters
½ tablespoon	7 milliliters
1 tablespoon (3 teaspoons)	15 milliliters
2 tablespoons (1 fluid ounce)	30 milliliters
¼ cup (4 tablespoons)	60 milliliters
⅓ cup	90 milliliters
½ cup (4 fluid ounces)	125 milliliters
⅔ cup	160 milliliters
¾ cup (6 fluid ounces)	180 milliliters
1 cup (16 tablespoons)	250 milliliters
1 pint (2 cups)	500 milliliters
1 quart (4 cups)	1 liter (about)

WEIGHT CONVERSIONS

U.S. Weight Measure	Metric Equivalent
½ ounce	15 grams
1 ounce	30 grams
2 ounces	60 grams
3 ounces	85 grams
¼ pound (4 ounces)	115 grams
½ pound (8 ounces)	225 grams
¾ pound (12 ounces)	340 grams
1 pound (16 ounces)	454 grams

OVEN TEMPERATURE CONVERSIONS

Degrees Fahrenheit	Degrees Celsius
200 degrees F	95 degrees C
250 degrees F	120 degrees C
275 degrees F	135 degrees C
300 degrees F	150 degrees C
325 degrees F	160 degrees C
350 degrees F	180 degrees C
375 degrees F	190 degrees C
400 degrees F	205 degrees C
425 degrees F	220 degrees C
450 degrees F	230 degrees C

BAKING PAN SIZES

U.S.	Metric
8 x 1½ inch round baking pan	20 x 4 cm cake tin
9 x 1½ inch round baking pan	23 x 3.5 cm cake tin
11 x 7 x 1½ inch baking pan	28 x 18 x 4 cm baking tin
13 x 9 x 2 inch baking pan	30 x 20 x 5 cm baking tin
2 quart rectangular baking dish	30 x 20 x 3 cm baking tin
15 x 10 x 2 inch baking pan	30 x 25 x 2 cm baking tin (Swiss roll tin)
9 inch pie plate	22 x 4 or 23 x 4 cm pie plate
7 or 8 inch springform pan	18 or 20 cm springform or loose bottom cake tin
9 x 5 x 3 inch loaf pan	23 x 13 x 7 cm or 2 lb narrow loaf or pate tin
1½ quart casserole	1.5 liter casserole
2 quart casserole	2 liter casserole

Index

Note: Page numbers in **bold** indicate recipe category lists.

We Have
EVERYTHING®
on Anything!

With more than 19 million copies sold, the Everything® series has become one of America's favorite resources for solving problems, learning new skills, and organizing lives. Our brand is not only recognizable—it's also welcomed.

The series is a hand-in-hand partner for people who are ready to tackle new subjects—like you!

For more information on the Everything® series, please visit *www.adamsmedia.com*

The Everything® list spans a wide range of subjects, with more than 500 titles covering 25 different categories:

Business	History	Reference
Careers	Home Improvement	Religion
Children's Storybooks	Everything Kids	Self-Help
Computers	Languages	Sports & Fitness
Cooking	Music	Travel
Crafts and Hobbies	New Age	Wedding
Education/Schools	Parenting	Writing
Games and Puzzles	Personal Finance	
Health	Pets	